The Late Eight

Second Edition

Ken M. Bleile, PhD

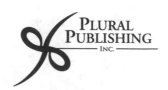

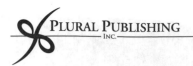

5521 Ruffin Road
San Diego, CA 92123

e-mail: info@pluralpublishing.com
Website: http://www.pluralpublishing.com

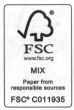

FSC
www.fsc.org
MIX
Paper from
responsible sources
FSC® C011935

Typeset in 11/13 Garamond by Flanagan's Publishing Services, Inc.
Printed in the United States of America by McNaughton & Gunn, Inc.

For permission to use material from this text, contact us by
Telephone: (866) 758-7251
Fax: (888) 758-7255
e-mail: permissions@pluralpublishing.com

*Every attempt has been made to contact the copyright holders for material orig-
inally printed in another source. If any have been inadvertently overlooked, the
publishers will gladly make the necessary arrangements at the first opportunity.*

Library of Congress Cataloging-in-Publication Data

Bleile, Ken Mitchell, author.
  The late eight / Ken M. Bleile.—Second edition.
      p. ; cm.
  Includes bibliographical references and index.
  ISBN-13: 978-1-59756-559-2 (alk. paper)
  ISBN-10: 1-59756-559-8 (alk. paper)
  I. Title.
  [DNLM: 1. Articulation Disorders—-diagnosis. 2. Articulation Disorders—therapy.
3. Language Development. 4. Speech Articulation Tests. WL 340.2]
  RC424.7
  616.85'5–dc23
                                                      2013025059

Contents

Preface

The first edition of *The Late Eight* was a book of all-purpose tools—the clinical equivalents of a carpenter's hammers, screwdrivers, bolts, paintbrushes, and ladder. The tools were designed to perform anything from an initial assessment to concluding a course of treatment, and were intended not to be "approach specific." Information on relative frequency or key environments, for example, is equally useful within a variety of phonological perspectives as in articulatory ones, or any other approach that might be developed.

This second edition of *The Late Eight* contains the same all-purpose clinical tools. Additionally, it describes how they may be employed within a specific clinical approach. To this purpose, the second edition contains a lengthy new chapter by Dr. Carlin Hageman outlining essential ideas about speech from a motor learning perspective. The DVD contains videos developed by Dr. Hageman that demonstrate aspects of a motor learning perspective.

Speech disorders in school-aged students deserve far more clinical and research attention than they presently receive. The second edition of *The Late Eight* furthers discussion of a newer and very exciting approach to the treatment of speech sound disorders in school-aged students. My hope is that future editions of the book will include more approaches, new and established, to help clinicians help students learn the verbal intricacies of the "late eight."

Ken Bleile
June, 2013

Contributor

Carlin Hageman, PhD
Professor and Head
ASHA Fellow
Communication Sciences and Disorders
University of Northern Iowa
Cedar Falls, IA
Chapter 12

Chapter One

Overview

Introduction

Six percent of all school-aged children experience difficulty acquiring the eight late-acquired sounds, and fully 92% of school-based clinicians have students with such speech problems on their caseloads (Shewan, 1988). Furthermore, because "the late eight" are more likely than early acquired sounds to be missing from the speech inventories of other languages, they often present special difficulties to nonnative speakers. In large urban areas such as New York City, one in four adults reports having difficulty speaking English (Bernstein, 2005). Across the United States, approximately 18% of children speak a language other than English at home.

Because speech problems affecting late-acquired sounds are the world's most frequently encountered communication disorder, every speech-language pathologist who works with school-aged students or nonnative English speakers should know how to treat them effectively and efficiently. In the first decades of our profession, numerous books, articles, chapters, and seminars helped a professional gain this knowledge. In more recent decades the flow of information and ideas has diminished to a bare trickle. As our contestant observed, the reason for this lessened interest is not because the frequency of this disorder has declined. Rather, the number of persons affected is larger due to increased native and immigrant populations.

Decreased attention to problems affecting such a large number of persons may reflect a change in professional emphasis, which has shifted to meet clinical demands presented by seemingly ever younger and more disabled children. Needs of an otherwise typically developing student who experiences difficulty saying a few late-acquired sounds are not often considered a high priority. Furthermore, a sense may exist among many professionals that ideas and materials to meet the needs of such a student were addressed long ago by Van Riper, McDonald, and other clinical pioneers (McDonald, 1964; Van Riper, 1978). Lastly, some have said (sometimes quietly, sometimes a little more loudly) that dealing with school-aged "artic" problems is simple and, well, boring.

Other Students Need Me More

School-aged students with "artic errors" as well as children and adults acquiring English as a nonnative language have needs that should not be marginalized. The numbers of such students is enormous and growing. Furthermore, although students with medical and extensive developmental needs demand clinical attention, one population of students should not be excluded for the sake of another. The sphere of clinical interests must include the entire range of students that are served, and a person should not be excluded from receiving service because of excellent potential for improvement. Furthermore, professional interest in children with more involved developmental needs does not preclude a similar interest in those on the other end of the severity continuum. Indeed, many clinicians find a balanced caseload is best, some with long-term developmental needs and others with more easily resolved problems.

All We Need to Know Was Written Long Ago

Nor is it the case everything needed to know to treat late-acquired sounds was written long ago. Although Van Riper's insights and those of other pioneers remain important and relevant, much has been learned in the intervening years, especially regarding language acquisition, second-language learning, inclusive practices, and motor learning. Ideas from those areas can and must shape and inform how a clinician thinks about treating late-acquired speech sounds. When these new ideas infuse clinical care, what a clinician does seems less like traditional articulation therapy and more like language therapy for speech disorders.

It's Simple

The belief that treating late-acquired sounds is simple may rise in part from an "artic" conception of speech disorders and partially from the organization of most university training programs. The first clinical experience of a student clinician typically is with a school-aged child with an error affecting a late-acquired sound, the rationale being that the procedures are straightforward "artic" and the behavior problems are fewer than with younger children (most times). This gives students the impression—a false one, the author believes—that such care is simple. Instead, it would be truer to say a student with errors affecting late-acquired sounds often shows excellent potential to improve, but to help a student achieve success a clinician must master complex speech and language therapy techniques while negotiating some challenging human issues. In any given day, for example, a clinician may facilitate pronunciation of [s] during a phonologic awareness activity, facilitate a third-grader's pronunciation of [l] as part of a class assignment on animals, and discuss with a teenager why therapy for multiple speech problems is needed. A clinician who believes such tasks are simple either is extremely gifted or may not have experienced the full range of challenges encountered when working with students with errors affecting late-acquired sounds.

It's Boring

Lastly, treatment for "the late eight" should not be boring either for a clinician or for a student. It is not always fun, fun, fun—but what type of valuable therapy is always fun, fun, fun? It is challenging work, requiring a solid understanding of speech, language, cognition, and learning. And, as in all clinical domains, a clinician must wrestle with such human variables as a student's motivation, focus, and personality. Challenging and rewarding? Yes. Boring? Only as boring or as exciting as the concepts and enthusiasm brought to it.

Resources for the Late Eight

Resources described in this chapter include 14 "tools of the trade" used to evaluate and treat late-acquired sounds. They include:

1. Definition
2. Acquisition
3. Relative frequency
4. Errors
5. Key environments
6. Metaphors
7. Touch cues
8. Initial screening
9. Screening for stimulability
10. Demonstrations
11. Phonetic placement and shaping techniques

12. Exercises
13. Language activities
14. Word lists

The chapter concludes with a description of resources on the accompanying DVD.

> ***Warning!***
>
> This chapter provides necessary background for using the resources. Most of the information, though important, is fairly dry to read.

1. Definition

What It Is: The definition is a prose description showing how a sound is produced, or, as in the case of sounds such as [s], [z], and [r], the several different ways it may be produced.

Its Uses: Typical uses of the definition include:

- Making an informed decision about how to teach a sound
- Explaining how a sound is produced to a student and family

Illustration: This is the definition of [s]:

> [s] is made in either of two ways. Some people produce [s] with the tongue tip up behind the upper front teeth, others say it with the tongue tip down behind the lower front teeth. Neither one is the "right way." Follow a student's lead in deciding which way to teach [s]. If a student appears to find it easier to say [s] with the tongue tip up, teach the sound that way; if a student appears to find it easier to say [s] with the tongue tip down, teach the sound that way. For both varieties of [s], the airstream is continuous and the vocal folds are apart.

A brief technical definition of the sound is also provided. This is the technical definition of [s]:

> [s] is voiceless alveolar fricative.

2. Acquisition

What It Is: Acquisition data show the ages at which 50% and 75% of children acquire a sound.

Its Uses: Acquisition data are widely used for two purposes:

- Deciding if a student's delay in acquisition of a sound is sufficient to warrant therapy
- Selecting between possible treatment sounds (some clinicians choose to treat earlier acquired sounds before treating later acquired ones)

Illustration: This is the acquisition data for [tʃ]:

> 50% of children acquire [tʃ] by 4;6 and 75% of children acquire [tʃ] by 5;6.

3. Relative Frequency

What It Is: Relative frequency is the relative frequency of occurrence of a sound in the language. The data source for relative frequency is Shriberg and Kwiatkowski (1983). The information is for consonants; vocalic [r] is excluded from the calculations.

Its Use: A typical use of information on relative frequency includes:

- Evaluating the contribution of a possible treatment sound on intelligibility (sounds with higher relative frequency are presumed to have greater influence on intelligibility than those that occur less frequently)

Illustration: This is the relative frequency for [z]:

> [z] is ranked fifth in relative frequency compared to the other late-acquired consonants. It ranks 15th in relative frequency compared to all other English consonants, and its percentage of occurrence compared to all English consonants is 3.0%.

4. Errors

What It Is: This resource shows the speech errors a student is likely to make when unable to pronounce a sound.

Its Uses: Knowledge of speech errors is widely used for at least two reasons:

- Identifying errors that may lead the student to be stigmatized socially
- Determining possible influence of an error on intelligibility (Errors with a relatively large effect on intelligibility include those found in the beginning of words, changes in place of pronunciation, and those involving sound deletions.)

Illustration: These are common [r] errors among students with errors affecting late-acquired sounds:

> The most common error is gliding—that is, [w] for [r]. Deletion of [r] after vowels and in consonant clusters also is a common error.

5. Key Environments

What It Is: Key environments describe phonetic environments in which a student is likely to pronounce a sound correctly. Key environments are "best bets" rather than absolute laws. Stated differently, a best bet is that a student will learn to pronounce a sound in a key environment rather than in another environment. Importantly, key environments for sounds overlap, with similarly pronounced sounds sharing similar key environments and less similarly pronounced sounds possessing fewer common key environments.

Its Use: Key environments are widely used for one important purpose:

- Helping decide in which phonetic environments to establish a treatment sound

Illustration: These are the key environments for [θ]

1. End of a syllable or word, as in *teeth*.
2. Before a high front vowel, as in *thin*.

6. Metaphors

What It Is: Metaphors provide a means to describe a sound.

Its Use: Metaphors are widely used for a single purpose:

- Providing the clinician and student a handy way to refer to a treatment sound

Illustration: These are possible metaphors for [z]:

Tongue placement:	Tongue tip sound	(tongue tip up or down)
	Bump sound little	(tongue tip up)
	Hill sound bottom	(tongue tip up)
	Teeth sound	(tongue tip down)
Fricative:	Snake sound	
	Long sound	
	Hissing sound	
Voicing:	Motor-on sound	
	Voice box on	
	Voice-on sound	
	Buzzing sound	
Word position:	Starting sound	Beginning of word
	End sound	End of word
	Sound friends	Consonant cluster

7. Touch Cues

What It Is: Touch cues draw attention to an aspect of a sound's production, typically the place of production.

Its Use: Typical uses of this resource include:

- Referring to a treatment sound through modalities (touch and sight) other than hearing
- Reminding a student how a treatment sound is produced

Illustration: This is the touch cue for [l]:

Tip of finger on the middle of the upper lip.

8. Initial Screening

What It Is: An initial screening helps determine if a student experiences difficulty pronouncing a late-acquired sound. It typically includes a spontaneous speech sample, and a short screening test that assesses possible errors at the word level in selected major phonetic contexts.

Its Use: Typical uses of this resource include:

- Helping decide if a student is a candidate for treatment
- Developing an initial hypothesis regarding types of errors made by a student
- Pretesting a student's ability to pronounce a sound

Illustration: This is the initial screening test for [ʃ]:

Instructions: I'm going to say some words. Please say the word after me.

Example: "Dog. Now you say it."

Word Beginning	*Student**
1. Shell	_____
2. Shutter	_____
3. Show	_____
4. Shrug	_____
5. Shrimp	_____
6. Shred	_____

Medial

7. Wishing	_____
8. Ocean	_____
9. Washer	_____

Final

10. Dish	_____
11. Crush	_____
12. Irish	_____
13. Harsh	_____
14. Marsh	_____
15. Borscht	_____

Suggestion: Transcribe an X if the sound is correct or, if incorrect, phonetically transcribe the error. Ignore errors produced elsewhere in the word.

Comments/Notes:

9. Screening for Stimulability

What It Is: A screening test for stimulability helps determine if a student is capable of pronouncing a sound. Stimulability is assessed in imitation, key environments, favorite words, and through phonetic placement and shaping. A sound may also be stimulable if it occurs in low frequency across a number of words; this is typically assessed through a spontaneous speech sample or through asking someone who knows the student well, perhaps a teacher or family member.

Its Use: The most typical use of this resource includes:

■ Selecting between possible treatment sounds (*Note*: Stimulability is a controversial topic. Some clinicians prefer to select a sound for which a student is stimulable, others prefer to select nonstimulable sounds.)

Illustration: This is the stimulability screening test for [tʃ]:

Imitation

1. **ch**ip _____

2. cat**ch** _____

Best Bet Environments

End of a syllable or word

1. [ɪ **tʃ**] _____

2. wat**ch** _____

After a high front vowel

1. bea**ch** _____

2. it**ch** _____

Favorite Words

Names of family members: _____

Favorite people, heroes, and activities: _____

Phonetic Placement

1. Ask the student to make the train sound, "choo choo."

Shaping

1. Instruct student to say, "Bet you" slowly.,
2. Next, instruct student to say, "Bet you" fast, resulting in the production of "Betcha."
3. If "betcha" doesn't work, repeat with, "Got you."

10. Demonstrations

What It Is: Demonstrations are formalized explanations showing how a sound is produced. Demonstrations can be simple or involved, some requiring no implements and others making use of a mirror and other tools. In general, simple demonstrations work best. If a clinician is going to put a hand in the student's mouth, all universal health care precautions should be followed.

Its Use: Typical uses of this resource include:

- Helping explain to a student how to pronounce a sound
- Focusing a student's attention on aspects of a sound pronounced incorrectly

Illustration: This is a simple demonstration of [s]:

Objects: Q-tip, peanut butter, or other favored food.

Instructions:

1. Instruct the student, "Please open your mouth."
2. Once the mouth is open, with Q-tip dab a little peanut butter or other favorite food on alveolar ridge (for tongue tip raised [s]) or behind lower front teeth (for tongue tip lowered [s]).
3. Ask the student to touch the food with the tongue tip.

11. Phonetic Placement and Shaping Techniques

What It Is: Phonetic placement and shaping techniques are procedures to teach sounds. Phonetic placement techniques entail instructing a student how to place the articulators to make a sound. Phonetic placement techniques are similar to demonstrations, the difference being that phonetic placement techniques require a production from a student and demonstrations do not. Shaping techniques rely on similarities between sounds to shape a sound a student can pronounce into one he or she cannot pronounce. Techniques presented in this book were culled from many sources, published and unpublished. The main published sources were books long out of print, most especially Nemoy and Davis (Nemoy & Davis, 1954). Unpublished sources include many talented and creative clinicians that the author has had the pleasure to interact with over the years.

> ### *What Phonetic Placement and Shaping Techniques Do*
> In essence, phonetic placement and shaping techniques make an unstimulable sound stimulable. Once stimulable, treatment then expands use of the sound in a student's speech.

Its Use: Typical uses of this resource include:

 Establishing a sound in a student's speech

Illustration: This is a phonetic placement technique for [θ], followed by technique for shaping vocalic [r] into consonantal [r]:

Phonetic Placement Technique for [θ]

Objects: feather or small piece of paper

Instructions:

1. Place a feather or small piece of paper in front of the student's mouth, about a half-inch to an inch from the tongue.
2. Instruct the student to blow air over the tongue to move the feather or paper, resulting in [θ].

Shaping Technique for [r]

Objects: None

Instructions:

1. Ask the student to say vocalic [r].
2. Next, ask the student to say vocalic [r] followed by [i] or some other vowel.
3. Instruct the student to say [i] several times as quickly as possible, resulting in vocalic [r] + [ri]. After [ri] is established, instruct the student to say vocalic [r] silently, resulting in [ri].

12. Speech Exercises

What It Is: Speech exercises help a student to gain experience pronouncing a treatment sound. Six different types of speech exercises are provided:

Imitation: The student repeats the word after you.

Minimal Pairs: The student says a word that contains the treatment sound, replaces the treatment sound to create a rhyming word, and then again says the word with the treatment sound.

Deletion: The student says a word that contains the treatment sound, says the same word with the treatment sound deleted, and then again says the word with the treatment sound added.

Self-Correction: The student says a word containing the treatment sound three times, self-correcting if errors in the treatment sound occur.

Old Way/New Way: The student says a word containing the treatment sound, pronouncing the treatment sound the new way, the old way, and then the new way again.

Similar Sound: The student says a word containing the treatment sound, replaces the treatment sound with the most similar sound the student can make, and then again says the word with the treatment sound.

Its Use: Typical uses of this resource include:

- Helping a student to master pronunciation of a late-acquired sound
- Helping a student learn to self-monitor and self-correct speech errors
- Focusing a student on the communication value of a late-acquired sound

Illustration: This is a possible use of two speech exercises in a treatment session.

Clinician: What is a word for ocean that starts with the snake sound?

Student: Sea.

Clinician: That's right. Do you remember how you used to say the *s* sound?

Student: th

Clinician: Good. Now say *sea* the new way, the old way, and then the new way again.

Student: Sea. Thea. Sea.

Clinician: Great. Now say *sea* three times, listening to yourself and trying to make the sound the new way.

Student: Sea. Sea. Sea.

13. *Language Activities*

What It Is: Language activities let a student practice a treatment sound in conversation and in school projects.

Its Use: Typical uses of this resource includes:

- Promoting generalization of a treatment sound to settings and persons outside the treatment session
- Helping to make a treatment sound a student's regular way of talking
- Practicing a treatment sound in linguistic contexts
- Promoting success on school assignments

Illustration: This is an awareness activity for [z] and a speech activity for [r], followed by an example showing ways in which an activity might be varied.

Awareness Activity for [z]

Ask a student to silently read a newspaper or story and then circle or write down words that contain [z].

Speech Activity for [r]

Give the student a printed story that has a sticker over words that contain [r]. Ask the student to read the story aloud and "to guess" at the words under the stickers. An easy alternative is to ask the student to say each stickered word the new way, the old way, and then the new way again.

14. *Word Lists*

What It Is: This book contains a list of approximately 4,000 different commonly found words containing late-acquired sounds. With very few exceptions, the words are short (one to two syllables) and easily pictured. The word lists for each sound are divided into major phonetic environments in which the sound occurs. Included in the word lists are lists of minimal pairs, deletions, and themes.

Its Use: This resource is used in many different ways, including:

- Developing pre- and posttests
- Practicing treatment sounds in isolated words
- Focusing a student on the linguistic role of a treatment sound
- Developing language-based activities

A Good Question

Someone may ask: Yes, but how do these word lists differ from those in the 40,000 words book—in addition to that book having 40,000 words and this book only having 4,000?

An Answer

The author has a well-worn copy of *40,000 Selected Words* (Blockcolsky, Frazer, & Frazer, 1987). The major differences between the word lists in that fine book and those in this book include:

- *The Late Eight* contains more than twice the number of words containing late-acquired sounds.
- The present book contains more short (one to three syllables), easily pictured words.
- Word lists in the present book are organized into minimal pairs, deletions, and themes.
- Word lists in the present book are organized according to phonetic environments frequently useful in treatment.

Illustration: The following is a sample of the entry for [s] at the beginning of words, followed by a theme for [l]:

Word List for [s]

Beginning of Words

Single Consonants	Deletions	Minimal Pairs
Sat	at	bat, mat, hat, cat, rat, pat
Salmon		
Sail	ale, ail	tail, pail, nail, veil, rail, whale, mail, jail
Salad		ballad
Sailboat		
Socks		fox, rocks, box
Soap		rope
Sew	O, oh	toe, row, hoe, no, bow, mow, go
Sun		fun, run, one, bun, gun
Sally	alley	tally
Silk	ilk	
Sea gull	eagle	

Theme for [l]

Northern Places	Deletions	Minimal Pairs
Chilly	hilly	Willy, silly, Billy
Elk		
Rudolph		
Sled	said	fled
Sled dog		
Sleigh bells		
Sleet	seat	fleet
Glacier		
Blizzard		
North Pole		
Cool		fool, tool, pool
Wolf	woof	
Wolves		
Sledding		
Sleigh	say	
Snowflake		

DVD

The accompanying DVD offers maximum portability and flexibility. Information in the DVD replicates much of the book, but in formats to download, print out, make into exercises, and to adapt as a clinician deems most suitable. The accompanying DVD includes the following printable materials for each late-acquired sound:

- A "Cheat Sheet"
- Initial Screening form
- Initial Stimulability Testing Form
- Demonstrations
- Phonetic placement and shaping exercises
- Shells for speech exercises
- Shells for language activities
- Complete word list
- Minimal pairs
- Deletions
- Themes

Summary

A speech sound disorder affecting late-acquired sounds is the world's most common type of communication problem. Resources contained in this book are "tools of the trade" to assist a clinician in evaluating and treating such speech disorders. The resources are flexible and can be used within a wide variety of therapeutic approaches and with a range of students, including children and adults, and both first and second language learners. The hope in assembling these resources is to help provide clinical care to the many students with this highly prevalent developmental difficulty.

References

Bernstein, N. (2005, January 19). Proficiency in English decreases over a decade. *New York Times.*

Blockcolsky, V., Frazer, J., & Frazer, D. (1987). *40,000 selected words.* San Antonio, TX: Communication Skills Builder.

McDonald, E. (1964). *A deep test of articulation.* Pittsburgh, PA: Stanwix House.

Nemoy, E., & Davis, S. (1954). *The correction of defective consonant sound.* Magnolia, MS: Expression.

Shewan, C. (1988). 1988 omnibus survey: Adaptation and progress in times of change. *Asha, 30,* 27–30.

Shriberg, L., & Kwiatkowski, J. (1983). Computer-assisted natural process analysis (NPA): Recent issues and data. In J. Locke (Ed.), *Seminars in Speech and Language, 4,* 397.

Van Riper, C. (1978). *Speech correction: Principles and methods* (6th ed.). Englewood Cliffs, NJ: Prentice-Hall.

Chapter Two
[θ]

Definition

[θ] is made with the tongue tip between the upper and lower front teeth. The airstream is a continuous hiss between the upper tongue and the upper teeth. The vocal folds are apart. The technical definition of [θ] is voiceless interdental fricative.

Acquisition

50% of children acquire [θ] by 4;6 and 75% of children acquire [θ] by 6;0.

Relative Frequency

[θ] is ranked 7th in relative frequency compared to the other late-acquired consonants. It ranks 21st in relative frequency compared to all other English consonants, and its percentage of occurrence compared to all English consonants is 0.9%.

Errors

[s] for [θ] is a common error, as is [f] for [θ]. Less common errors for [θ] among school-aged students is [t] or [p] for [θ].

Key Environments

End of a syllable or word, as in *teeth*
Before a high front vowel, as *thin*

Possible Metaphors

Select metaphors based on the aspect of speech that is the focus of therapy.

Tongue placement: Tongue tip sound

Fricative: Leaky tire sound
                    Long sound
                    Hissing sound

Voicing: Motor off
                    Voice off
                    Not a buzzing sound
                    Voice box off

Touch Cue

Finger in front of lips.

Instructions

Place the student's finger in the middle of the front of the lips.

Initial Screening Test for [θ]

Student's Name: _____

Date: _____

Referral: _____

Instructions: Say to the student, "I'm going to say some words. Please say the words after me."
Example: "Dog. Now you say it."

Word	Student*
Beginning	
1. Thigh	_____
2. Thunder	_____
3. Thorn	_____
4. Threw	_____
5. Thriller	_____
6. Throne	_____
Medial	
7. Nothing	_____
8. Python	_____
9. Without	_____
Final	
10. Bath	_____
11. Oath	_____
12. Teeth	_____
13. Sixth	_____
14. Ninth	_____
15. North	_____

*Suggestion: Transcribe an X if the sound is correct or, if incorrect, phonetically transcribe the error. Ignore errors produced elsewhere in the word.

Comments/Notes:

Stimulability Tests for [θ]

Student's Name: _____

Date: _____

Referral: _____

Imitation

1. **Th**umb   _____
2. Too**th**   _____

Best Bet Environments

End of a syllable or word

1. tee**th**   _____
2. [i**θ**]   _____

Before a high front vowel

1. **th**in   _____
2. [**θ**i]   _____

Favorite Words

Names of family members: _____

Favorite people, heroes, and activities: _____

Phonetic Placement   _____

1. Ask the student to place the tongue between the upper and lower teeth.
2. Instruct the student to put his or her hand in front of the mouth, and blow through the teeth to feel the airflow.

Shaping [θ] from [s]   _____

1. Demonstrate the difference between the place of production for [s] and the place of production for [θ].
2. Next, instruct the student to say /s/ while moving his or her tongue to rest between the upper and lower teeth, resulting in [θ].

Notes/Comments:

Demonstrations for [θ]

Place: Interdental

First Method _____

Object: Tongue depressor

Instructions:

1. Instruct the student, "Please stick out your tongue."
2. Once the tongue is out, gently close the student's mouth. If the tongue is sticking out too far, gently push it back with a tongue depressor.

Second Method _____

Objects: Tongue depressor or stick of candy or other favored food

Instructions:

1. Place a tongue depressor or piece of food in front of the student's mouth, about half an inch before the lips.
2. Instruct the student, "Please touch it with your tongue."
3. While the student touches the tongue depressor or food with the tongue tip, gently close the student's mouth.
4. Instruct the student, "Now pull your tongue back just a little until I say stop."

Manner: Fricative

First Method _____

Objects: Strip of paper or a feather

Instructions:

1. Place a strip of paper, a feather, or the student's hand held in front of your mouth while you produce several long voiceless fricatives.
2. Draw attention to the "hissing" quality and continuous nature of the sounds.

Second Method

Objects: A small paper flower on end of a pencil

Instructions:

Tape a small paper flower on the end of a pencil and encourage the student to move the flower in the wind.

Third Method

Objects: None

Instructions:

Run your finger or the student's finger down the student's arm while making several long voiceless fricatives to demonstrate the "hissing" quality and length of fricatives.

Voicing: Voiceless

First Method

Objects: None

Instructions:

Instruct the student to listen to and identify the difference between a voiceless and voiced [a].

Second Method

Objects: None

Instructions:

Place the student's hands over the ears and instruct him or her to hum, which heightens the sensation of vocal cord vibration.

Third Method

Objects: None

Instructions:

If the student is able to produce a voiced and voiceless fricative, ask him or her to cover the ears and make these sounds. Alternatively, ask the student to make [h] and [a].

Fourth Method

Objects: None

Instructions:

You and the student place one hand on your throat and the other on the student's throat while making voiced and voiceless sounds together, telling each other when the voicing goes on and off.

Fifth Method

Objects: Pencil, small piece of paper or small paper flower

Instructions:

If the student is able to produce a pair of voiced and voiceless oral stops, attach a small piece of paper or a paper flower to the end of a tongue depressor or pencil and ask the student to "make the paper (or flower) move." The paper is more likely to move when a voiceless consonant is produced than when a voiced consonant is produced (be careful in providing instructions to the student, however, because a strongly articulated voiced oral stop will also move the flower).

Phonetic Placement and Shaping Techniques for [θ]

Phonetic Placement Techniques

Both these simple phonetic placement methods focus on tongue placement (tongue between the teeth) and airflow (air over the tongue).

First Method

Objects: feather or small piece of paper

Instructions:

1. Place a feather or small piece of paper in front of the student's mouth, about one-half inch to an inch from the tongue.
2. Ask the student to blow air over the tongue to move the feather or paper, resulting in [θ].

Second Method

Objects: Tongue depressor and Q-tip

Instructions:

1. Place a tongue depressor in front of the student's mouth, instructing the student to touch the depressor with his or her tongue tip.
2. When the student's tongue is out, gently push up the student's lower jaw so that his or her teeth and tongue come into contact.
3. Instruct the student to blow air over the tongue. If the student produces an interdental [t], gently insert a Q-tip between the student's tongue tip and upper teeth to create a sufficiently broad opening to allow continuous airflow, resulting in [θ].

Shaping Exercises

(θ) from (f)

This method is for a student with a well-established [f].

Objects: None

Instructions:

1. Demonstrate the difference between the places of production for [f] and [θ].
2. Ask the student to say [f] while moving the tongue to lie between the upper and lower front teeth, resulting in [θ]. (*Note*: To facilitate [ð], develop from [v].

(θ) from (s)

This method approaches [θ] from the opposite direction as the first method: rather than from slightly anterior [f], this method approaches [θ] from slightly posterior [s].

Objects: None

Instructions:

1. Demonstrate the difference between the place of production for [s] and the place of production for [θ].
2. Next, instruct the student to say [s] while moving the tongue to lie between the upper and lower front teeth, resulting in [θ]. (*Note*: To facilitate the [ð], develop from [z].

Shell for Speech Exercises

Student's Name: _____

Date: _____

Treatment Sound: _____

Word List: Student Responses:

                                                   1. _____

     2. _____

     3. _____

     4. _____

     5. _____

     6. _____

     7. _____

     8. _____

     9. _____

    10. _____

Total Correct: _____ / _____

Comments:

Imitation

Student's Name: _____

Date: _____

Treatment Sound: _____

Goal: Have the student repeat the word after you.

Instructions to Student: "You are going to hear a word with our sound. Please say it after me. Here's an example. I say *sat*, and then you say *sat*."

Word List:	Student Responses:
Thin	1. _____
Thumper	2. _____
Thick	3. _____
Thief	4. _____
Thumb	5. _____
Thank you	6. _____
Thigh	7. _____
Thunder	8. _____
Thorn	9. _____
Thumbtack	10. _____

Total Correct: _____ / _____

Comments:

Minimal Pairs

Student's Name _____

Date: _____

Treatment Sound: _____

Goal: Have the student first say the word with the treatment sound, then say the rhyming word, and then say the word with the treatment sound.

Instructions to Student: "You are going to hear a word that begins with our sound. Please say the word, then replace our sound with another sound to make the word have a different meaning, and then say the word with our sound again. Here's an example. I say *seal*. You say *seal*, then change [s] to [w] to make *wheel*, and then say *seal* again. Like this: *Seal. Wheel. Seal.*"

Word List:		Student Responses:
Thin	chin	1. _____
Thor	soar	2. _____
Third	word	3. _____
Thumper	jumper	4. _____
Thatch	hatch	5. _____
Think	pink	6. _____
Thick	sick	7. _____
Thief	chief	8. _____
Thumb	gum	9. _____
Thigh	bye	10. _____

Total Correct: _____ / _____

Comments:

Deletion

Student's Name _____

Date: _____

Treatment Sound: _____

Goal: Have the student first say the word with the treatment sound, then without the treatment sound, and then with the treatment sound.

Instructions to Student: "You are going to hear word with our sound. Please say the word, and then say it with our sound deleted, and then say it with our sound included. Here's an example. I say *red*. You say *red*, then *Ed*, then *red*. Like this: *Red. Ed. Red*."

Word List:		Student Responses:
Thin	in	1. _____
Thick	ick	2. _____
Thumb	um	3. _____
Thigh	I, eye	4. _____
Thug	ugh	5. _____
Thor	or	6. _____
Thaw	awe	7. _____
Thought	ought	8. _____
Think	ink	9. _____
Theory	eerie	10. _____

Total Correct: _____ / _____

Comments:

Self-Correction

Student's Name _____

Date: _____

Treatment Sound: _____

Goal: Have the student say the word three times, self correcting if errors in the treatment sound occur.

Instructions to Student: "You are going to hear a word with our sound. Please say the word three times, listening to how you say our sound and changing it to make it correctly if you say it incorrectly. Here's an example. I say *cheese*, and then you say *cheese* three times, listening to how you say our sound and changing it to make it correctly if you say it incorrectly. Like this: *Cheese. Cheese. Cheese.*

Word List: **Student Responses:**

Thin   1. _____

Thumper   2. _____

Thick   3. _____

Thief   4. _____

Thumb   5. _____

Thank you   6. _____

Thigh   7. _____

Thunder   8. _____

Thorn   9. _____

Thumbtack   10. _____

Total Correct: _____ / _____

Comments:

Old Way/New Way

Student's Name _____

Date: _____

Treatment Sound: _____

Goal: Have the student say the word the new way, the old way, and then the new way again.

Instructions to Student: "You are going to hear a word with our sound. Please say the word, then say it the old way you used to say our sound, and then say it the new way you say our sound. Here's an example. I say *thin*. You say *thin*, then **in*, and then *thin*. Like this: *Thin. *in. Thin.*

Note: Replace * with the way the student used to say the sound.

Word List:	Student Responses:
Thin	1. _____
Thumper	2. _____
Thick	3. _____
Thief	4. _____
Thumb	5. _____
Thank you	6. _____
Thigh	7. _____
Thunder	8. _____
Thorn	9. _____
Thumbtack	10. _____

Total Correct: _____ / _____

Comments:

Similar Sound

Student's Name _____

Date: _____

Treatment Sound: _____

Goal: Have the student first say the word with the treatment sound, then with the most similar sound the student can make, and then with the treatment sound again.

Instructions to Student: "You are going to hear a word with our sound. Please say the word, then replace our sound with *__, and then say the word with our sound. Here's an example. I say *sun*. You say *sun*, then **un*, and then *sun* again. Like this: *Sun*. **un*. *Sun*.

Note: Replace * with a sound the student can pronounce that is phonetically similar to the treatment sound.

Word List: Student Responses:

Thin   1. _____

Thumper   2. _____

Thick   3. _____

Thief   4. _____

Thumb   5. _____

Thank you   6. _____

Thigh   7. _____

Thunder   8. _____

Thorn   9. _____

Thumbtack   10. _____

Total Correct: _____ / _____

Comments:

Complete Word List for [θ]

Beginning of Words

Single Consonants	Deletions	Minimal Pairs
Thin	in	chin, pin
Thumper		jumper, bumper
Thick	ick	sick, kick, tick, pick, wick, lick
Thief		chief, beef, leaf
Thumb	um	gum
Thank you		
Thigh	I, eye	bye, high, pie, tie
Thunder		sunder
Thorn		corn, torn, horn, worn
Thumbtack		
Thong		long, song
Thighbone		my bone
Thimble		nimble, cymbal
Thug	ugh	bug, hug
Thelma		Selma
Thebes		dweebs
Thorny		corny
Thorax		Borax
Third		bird, word, nerd, heard
Thor	or	soar, core, shore, floor
Thanks		banks
Thursday		
Third base		
Thirty		dirty
Thoreau		
Thaw	awe	paw, saw
Things		
Thinnest		
Thought	ought	caught, bought
Thousand		
Thirteen		
Third world		
Thermal		
Thirsty		
Thicket		picket, wicket
Think	ink	rink, wink, pink
Thermos		

Single Consonants	Deletions	Minimal Pairs
Theme song		
Thebe		dweeb
Thoughtful		
Thatch		batch, hatch
Theory	eerie	dearie
Thorough		burrow
Thirst		burst, nursed
Thistle		missile

Consonant Clusters	Deletions	Minimal Pairs
Three		tree
Throw	row	
Thrill	rill	
Throttle		
Thrift shop		
Thread	read	tread
Throat	wrote	
Threw	rue	true, crew
Throw rug		
Thriller		
Throne	roan	grown, prone
Thrifty		
Throwing	rowing	
Threshold		
Throng	wrong	prong
Thirsty		
Thrive		
Thrash	rash	crash, brash, lash
Through	rue	grew, true, crew
Thrush	rush	brush, crush
Threat		
Thrust	rust	crust
Throb	rob	

Medial

Single Consonants

Nothing	Toothpick	Author
South Seas	Martha	Nathan
Something	Toothpaste	Kathy
Playthings	Bathroom	Athens
Earthquake	Toothless	Carthage
Athlete	Bathmat	Earthling
Mouthwash	Toothbrush	Gothic
Panther	Python	Fifth grade
Playthings	Without	Bathtub
Southpaw	Toothache	Mathew

Consonant Clusters

Heartthrob	Fourth grade	North Star
Monthly	Jethro	Anthrax
Swarthmore	Darth Mal	Cutthroat
North Pole	Darth Vader	
Bathrobe	Bathroom	

All Environments

Mouthwash	Earthquake	Athens
Heartthrob	Athlete	Fourth grade
Nothing	North Star	Toothless
Darth Mal	Something	North Pole
Panther	Author	Bathmat
Jethro	Cutthroat	Monthly
Bathroom	Nathan	Fifth grade
Playthings	Kathy	Bathtub
Toothpick	South Seas	Toothache
Anthrax	Darth Vader	Gothic
Python	Carthage	Mathew
Martha	Earthling	Toothbrush
Swarthmore	Toothpaste	Bathrobe

Ends of Words

Single Consonants	*Deletions*
Mammoth	
Bath	baa
Oath	oh
Dishcloth	
Ruth	rue
Teeth	tea
Babe Ruth	
Steam bath	
Macbeth	
Sith	
Goldsmith	
Sloth	slaw
Keith	key
Sweet tooth	
Bike Path	
Swath	
Birdbath	
Tooth	two
Sleuth	slew
Math	
Phone booth	
Kenneth	
Plymouth	
Faith	fey, Fay
South	sow
Blacksmith	
Sheath	she
Path	
Faith	Fay, fey
Mouth	Mao
Cheesecloth	
Beth	
Breath	
Myth	
Broth	braw
Booth	boo
Death	
Wreath	

Consonant Clusters

Consonant Clusters	Deletions
Fourth	four
Fifth	
Sixth	six
Seventh	seven
Eighth	eight
Ninth	nine
Tenth	ten
Eleventh	eleven
Twelfth	
North	nor
Warmth	warm

Themes for [θ]

Themes

Teeth Brushing	Actions
Bath Time	Numbers and Days
Star Wars Villains	Days of Christmas
Around the Home	Directions
It's a Job	People and Places
Nature	

Teeth Brushing

Teeth Brushing	Deletions	Minimal Pairs
Toothache		
Toothless		
Teeth	T, tea	wreath, Keith
Mouth	Mao	
Breath		
Thirst		burst, nursed
Sweet tooth		
Tooth	two	
Toothbrush		
Thirsty		
Mouthwash		
Toothpick		
Toothpaste		

Bath Time	Deletions	Minimal Pairs
Thumb		gum
Thigh	I, eye	bye, high, pie, tie
Mouth		
Throat	wrote	
Bathmat		
Bathtub		
Bathrobe		
Bathroom		
Bath	baa	
Playthings		

Star Wars Villains	Deletions	Minimal Pairs
Sith		
Darth Mal		
Darth Vader		
Throne	roan	grown, prone
Threat		

Around the Home	Deletions	Minimal Pairs
Bathmat		
Bathtub		
Thermos		
Threshold		
Bathrobe		
Bathroom		
Thimble		nimble, cymbal
Throw rug		
Thumbtack		
Mouthwash		
Playthings		
Toothpick		
Broth	bra	
Thread	read	tread
Toothpaste		
Thong		long, song

It's a Job	**Deletions**	**Minimal Pairs**
Athlete		
Author		
Sleuth	slew	
Blacksmith		
Cutthroat		
Thief		chief, beef, leaf
Thug		bug, hug

Nature	**Deletions**	**Minimal Pairs**
Path		
Thistle		missile
Thatch		batch, hatch
Thrush	rush	brush, crush
Thicket		picket
Mammoth		
Sloth	slaw	
Bike Path		
Thaw	awe	saw, paw
Panther		
Earthquake		
Python		
Thorny		corny
Thunder		
Thorn		corn, torn, horn, worn

Actions	**Deletions**	**Minimal Pairs**
Throwing	rowing	
Thrive		
Think	ink	rink, wink, pink
Thrash	rash	crash, brash, lash
Threaten		
Thrust	rust	crust
Throb	rob	
Throw	row	crow, pro
Threw	rue	true

Numbers and Days	Deletions	Minimal Pairs
Three	tree	
Fourth	four	
Fourth grade		
Tenth	ten	
Monthly		
Thursday		
Third		bird, word, nerd, heard
Third base		
Thirty		dirty
Thousand		
Sixth grade		
Fifth grade		
Thirteen		
Third world		

Days of Christmas	Deletions	Minimal Pairs
Third		bird, word, nerd, heard
Fourth	four	
Fifth		
Sixth	six	
Seventh	seven	
Eighth	eight	
Ninth	nine	
Tenth	ten	
Eleventh	eleven	
Twelfth		

Directions	Deletions	Minimal Pairs
North	nor	
South	sow	

People and Places	Deletions	Minimal Pairs
North Star		
Jethro		
Thumper		jumper, bumper
Swarthmore		
North Pole		
South Seas		
Faith	fey, Fay	
Babe Ruth		
Ruth	rue	
Thebe		dweeb
Mathew		
Thebes		dweebs
Beth		
Athens		
Nathan		
Kathy		
Carthage		
Martha		
Nathan		
Macbeth		
Goldsmith		
Keith		
Kenneth		
Plymouth		
Thelma		Selma
Thor	or	soar, core, shore, floor
Thoreau		

Chapter Three

[ð]

Definition

[ð] is made with the tongue tip between the upper and lower front teeth. The airstream is a continuous hiss between the upper tongue and the upper teeth. The vocal folds are together. The technical definition of [ð] is voiced interdental fricative.

Acquisition

50% of children acquire [ð] by 4;6 and 75% of children acquire [ð] by 5;6.

Relative Frequency

[ð] is ranked 4th in relative frequency compared to the other late-acquired consonants. It ranks 11th in relative frequency compared to all other English consonants, and its percentage of occurrence compared to all English consonants is 4.1%.

Errors

[d] for [ð] is a common error. A less common error among school-aged students is [b] for [ð].

Key Environments

Between vowels, as in *weather*
Before a high front vowel, as in *these*

Possible Metaphors

Select metaphors based on the aspect of speech that is the focus of therapy.

Tongue placement: Tongue tip sound

Fricative: Leaky tire sound
                    Long sound
                    Hissing sound

Voicing: Motor on
                    Buzzing sound
                    Voice box on sound

Touch Cue

Finger in front of lips.

Instructions

Place the student's finger in the middle of the front of the lips.

Initial Screening Test for [ð]

Student's Name: _____

Date: _____

Referral: _____

Instructions: Say to the student, "I'm going to say some words. Please say the words after me."
Example: "Dog. Now you say it."

Word	Student*
Beginning	
1. This	_____
2. Them	_____
3. Then	_____
4. The	_____
Medial	
5. Clothing	_____
6. Weather	_____
7. Father	_____
8. Feather	_____
Final	
9. Breathe	_____
10. Teethe	_____
11. Sheathe	_____
12. Soothe	_____

Suggestion: Transcribe an X if the sound is correct or, if incorrect, phonetically transcribe the error. Ignore errors produced elsewhere in the word.

Comments/Notes:

Stimulability Tests for [ð]

Student's Name: _____

Date: _____

Referral: _____

Imitation

1. <u>th</u>e   _____

2. mo<u>th</u>er   _____

Best Bet Environments

Between vowels

1. wea<u>th</u>er   _____

2. ei<u>th</u>er   _____

Before a high front vowel

1. <u>th</u>ese   _____

2. <u>th</u>is   _____

Favorite Words

Names of family members: _____

Favorite people, heroes, and activities: _____

Phonetic Placement   _____

1. Demonstrate placing the tongue between the upper and lower teeth.

2. Instruct the student to put his or her hand in front of the mouth, and blow through the teeth to feel the airflow with the voice box turned on.

Shaping (ð) from (z)   _____

1. Demonstrate the difference between the place of production for [z] and the place of production for [ð].

2. Next, instruct the student to say [z] while moving his or her tongue to rest between his or her upper and lower teeth, resulting in [ð].

Notes/Comments:

Demonstrations for [ð]

Place: Interdental

First Method _____

Object: Tongue depressor

Instructions:

1. Instruct the student, "Please stick out your tongue."
2. Once the tongue is out, gently close the student's mouth. If the tongue is sticking out too far, gently push it back with a tongue depressor.

Second Method _____

Objects: Tongue depressor or stick of candy or other favored food.

Instructions:

1. Place a tongue depressor or piece of food in front of the student's mouth, about half an inch before the lips.
2. Instruct the student, "Please touch it with your tongue."
3. While the student touches the tongue depressor or food with the tongue tip, gently close the student's mouth.
4. Instruct the student, "Now pull your tongue back just a little until I say stop."

Manner: Fricative

First Method _____

Objects: Strip of paper or a feather

Instructions:

1. Place a strip of paper, a feather, or the student's hand held in front of your mouth while you produce several long voiceless fricatives.
2. Draw attention to the "hissing" quality and continuous nature of the sounds.

Second Method

Objects: A small paper flower on end of a pencil

Instructions: Tape a small paper flower on the end of a pencil and encourage the student to move the flower in the wind.

Third Method

Objects: None

Instructions: Run your finger or the student's finger down the student's arm while making several long voiceless fricatives to demonstrate the "hissing" quality and length of fricatives.

Voicing: Voiced

First Method

Objects: None

Instructions: Instruct the student to listen to and identify the difference between a voiceless and voiced [a].

Second Method

Objects: None

Instructions: Place the student's hands over the ears and instruct him or her to hum, which heightens the sensation of vocal cord vibration.

Third Method

Objects: None

Instructions: If the student is able to produce a voiced and voiceless fricative, ask him or her to cover the ears and make these sounds. Alternatively, the student is asked to make [h] and [a].

Fourth Method _____

Objects: None

Instructions: You and the student place one hand on your throat and the other on the student's throat while making voiced and voiceless sounds together, telling each other when the voicing goes on and off.

Fifth Method _____

Objects: Pencil, small piece of paper or small paper flower

Instructions: If the student is able to produce a pair of voiced and voiceless oral stops, attach a small piece of paper or a paper flower to the end of a tongue depressor or pencil and ask the student to "make the paper (or flower) move." The paper is more likely to move when a voiceless consonant is produced than when a voiced consonant is produced (be careful in providing instructions to the student, however, because a strongly articulated voiced oral stop will also move the flower).

Phonetic Placement and Shaping Techniques for [ð]

To facilitate [ð], follow the steps for [θ] but also use demonstrations to instruct the student to turn on the voice box.

Shell for Speech Exercises

Student's Name: _____

Date: _____

Treatment Sound: _____

Word List: **Student Responses:**

1. _____

2. _____

3. _____

4. _____

5. _____

6. _____

7. _____

8. _____

9. _____

10. _____

Total Correct: _____ / _____

Comments:

Imitation

Student's Name: _____

Date: _____

Treatment Sound: _____

Goal: Have the student repeat the word after you.

Instructions to Student: "You are going to hear a word with our sound. Please say it after me. Here's an example. I say *sat*, and then you say *sat*."

Word List:	Student Responses:
That	1. _____
This	2. _____
Them	3. _____
Then	4. _____
The Hague	5. _____
Their	6. _____
Those	7. _____
These	8. _____
They	9. _____
There	10. _____

Total Correct: _____/_____

Comments:

Minimal Pairs

Student's Name: _____

Date: _____

Treatment Sound: _____

Goal: Have the student first say the word with the treatment sound, then say the rhyming word, and then say the word with the treatment sound.

Instructions to Student: "You are going to hear a word that begins with our sound. Please say the word, then replace our sound with another sound to make the word have a different meaning, and then say the word with our sound again. Here's an example. I say *seal*. You say *seal*, then change [s] to [w] to make *wheel*, and then say *seal* again. Like this: *Seal. Wheel. Seal.*"

Word List:		Student Responses:
They	hay	1. _____
Than	can	2. _____
Though	toe	3. _____
Their	bear	4. _____
Those	nose	5. _____
These	bees	6. _____
There	bear	7. _____
That	sat	8. _____
Then	Ben	9. _____
They	bay	10. _____

Total Correct: _____ / _____

Comments:

Deletion

Student's Name: _____

Date: _____

Treatment Sound: _____

Goal: Have the student first say the word with the treatment sound, then without the treatment sound, and then with the treatment sound.

Instructions to Student: "You are going to hear a word with our sound. Please say the word, and then say it with our sound deleted, and then say it with our sound included. Here's an example. I say *red*. You say *red*, then *Ed*, then *red*. Like this: *Red. Ed. Red.*"

Word List:		Student Responses:
They	A	1. _____
Than	Ann	2. _____
Though	O	3. _____
Their	air	4. _____
Those	Os	5. _____
These	ease	6. _____
There	air	7. _____
That	at	8. _____
Then	N	9. _____
They	A	10. _____

Total Correct: _____ / _____

Comments:

Self-Correction

Student's Name: _____

Date: _____

Treatment Sound: _____

Goal: Have the student say the word three times, self-correcting if errors in the treatment sound occur.

Instructions to Student: "You are going to hear a word with our sound. Please say the word three times, listening to how you say our sound and changing it to make it correctly if you say it incorrectly. Here's an example. I say *cheese*, and then you say *cheese* three times, listening to how you say our sound and changing it to make it correctly if you say it incorrectly. Like this: *Cheese. Cheese. Cheese.*"

Word List:	Student Responses:
That	1. _____
This	2. _____
Them	3. _____
Then	4. _____
The Hague	5. _____
Their	6. _____
Those	7. _____
These	8. _____
They	9. _____
There	10. _____

Total Correct: _____ / _____

Comments:

Old Way/New Way

Student's Name: _____

Date: _____

Treatment Sound: _____

Goal: Have the student say the word the new way, the old way, and then the new way again.

Instructions to Student: "You are going to hear a word with our sound. Please say the word, then say it the old way you used to say our sound, and then say it the new way you say our sound. Here's an example. I say *thin*. You say *thin*, then **in*, and then *thin*. Like this: *Thin. *in. Thin.*"

Note: Replace * with the way the student used to say the sound.

Word List:	Student Responses:
That	1. _____
This	2. _____
Them	3. _____
Then	4. _____
The Hague	5. _____
Their	6. _____
Those	7. _____
These	8. _____
They	9. _____
There	10. _____

Total Correct: _____ / _____

Comments:

Similar Sound

Student's Name: _____

Date: _____

Treatment Sound: _____

Goal: Have the student first say the word with the treatment sound, then with the most similar sound the student can make, and then with the treatment sound again.

Instructions to Student: "You are going to hear a word with our sound. Please say the word, then replace our sound with _____*, and then say the word with our sound. Here's an example. I say *sun*. You say *sun*, then **un*, and then *sun* again. Like this: *Sun. *un. Sun.*"

Note: Replace * with a sound the student can pronounce that is phonetically similar to the treatment sound.

Word List:	Student Responses:
That	1. _____
This	2. _____
Them	3. _____
Then	4. _____
The Hague	5. _____
Their	6. _____
Those	7. _____
These	8. _____
They	9. _____
There	10. _____

Total Correct: _____ / _____

Comments:

Complete Word List for [ð]

Beginning of Words

Single Consonants	Deletions	Minimal Pairs
That	at	sat, mat, cat, fat, bat
This		kiss, hiss
Them	M	REM
Then	N	Ben, hen, pen, men
The Hague		
Their	air	bear, share, care, fair
Those	Os	nose, toes, bows
These	ease	bees, cheese, knees
They	A	hay, bay, say, day, gray
There	air	bear, share, care, fair
The	a	
Than	Ann	can, man, fan, ran
Though	O, oh	toe, bow, go, show, no

Medial

Single Consonants

Clothing	Slither	Northern
Weather	Mother	Earthquake
Father	Leather	Brother
Heather	Breathing	Bathrobe
Teething	Arthur	Bathing
Bather	Feather	Smoothest

Consonant Clusters

—

End of Words

Single Consonants	Deletions
Breathe	Bree
Teethe	tea
Sheathe	she
Soothe	Sue
Bathe	bay
Unsheathe	
Smooth	
Clothe	
Scythe	
Sun bathe	

Themes for [ð]

Themes

Nature	The Body
People and Places	Grammatic Words
Bath Time	Family

Nature	Deletions	Minimal Pairs
Sun bathe		
Earthquake		
Slither		
Leather		feather, weather, heather
Weather		feather, leather
Feather		weather, heather, leather
Heather		feather, weather, leather
Northern		

People and Places	Deletions	Minimal Pairs
The Hague		
Arthur		
Heather		feather, weather, leather

Bath Time	**Deletions**	**Minimal Pairs**
Bathe	bay	
Bather		
Bathing		
Bathrobe		
Clothe		
Clothing		
Bather	Bayer	

The Body	**Deletions**	**Minimal Pairs**
Breathe	Bree	
Breathing		
Teethe	T, tea	
Teething		

Grammatic Words	**Deletions**	**Minimal Pairs**
That	at	sat, mat, cat, fat, bat
This		kiss, hiss
Them	M	
Then	N	Ben, hen, pen, men
Their	air	bear, air, share, care, fair
Those		nose, toes, bows
These	ease	bees, cheese, knees
They	A	hay, bay, say, day, gray
The	a	
Than	Ann	can, man, fan, ran
Though	O, oh	toe, bow, go, show, no

Family	**Deletions**	**Minimal Pairs**
Brother		mother, other
Father		bother
Mother		other, mother

Chapter Four

[s]

Definition

[s] is made in either of two ways. Some people produce [s] with the tongue tip up behind the upper front teeth, others say [s] with the tongue tip down behind the lower front teeth. Neither one is the "right way." Follow the student's lead in deciding which way to teach [s]. If the student appears to find it easier to say [s] with the tongue tip up, teach the sound that way; if the student appears to find it easier to say [s] with the tongue tip down, teach the sound that way. For both varieties of [s], the airstream is continuous and the vocal folds are apart. The technical definition of [s] is voiceless alveolar fricative.

Acquisition

50% of children acquire [s] by 3;6 and 75% of children acquire [s] by 6;0.

Relative Frequency

[s] is ranked 1st in relative frequency compared to the other late-acquired consonants. It ranks 3rd in relative frequency compared to all other English consonants, and its percentage of occurrence compared to all English consonants is 7.1%.

Errors

A common error for [s] is Lisping. During Lisping [s] is pronounced with the tongue tip between the teeth as for [θ]. Another common error for [s] is using the tongue blade instead of the tongue tip, which is sometimes called Bladed [s]. A third common error is Lateralizing, in which instead of air flowing over the top of the tongue it flows over the sides of the tongue as for an [l].

Key Environments

End of a syllable or word, as in *bus*
Before a high front vowel, as in *see*
After [t] and before [i], as in *pizza*
After a [t] occurring in the same syllable, as in *beats*

Possible Metaphors

Select metaphors based on the aspect of speech that is the focus of therapy.

Tongue placement:	Tongue tip sound,
	Bmp sound (tongue tip up)
	Little hill sound (tongue tip up)
	Lower teeth sound (tongue tip down)
Fricative:	Snake sound
	Long sound
	Hissing sound
Voicing:	Motor off
	Voice off
	Not a buzzing sound
	Voice box off

Touch Cue

Finger on the corner of the mouth (finger up for tongue tip raised sound or finger down for tongue tip down sound).

Instruction:

Place the student's finger in the corner of the lips, and remind the student to keep upper and lower teeth close together.

Initial Screening Test for [s]

Student's Name: _____

Date: _____

Referral: _____

Instructions: Say to the student, "I'm going to say some words. Please say the words after me."
Example: "Dog. Now you say it."

Word	Student*	Word	Student*
Beginning			
1. Soap	_____	6. Skirt	_____
2. Sew	_____	7. Smell	_____
3. Sun	_____	8. Slap	_____
4. Sting	_____	9. Strap	_____
5. Spicy	_____		
Medial			
10. Acid	_____		
11. Messy	_____		
12. Icing	_____		
Final			
13. Dice	_____	17. Husk	_____
14. Moose	_____	18. Toast	_____
15. House	_____	19. Fierce	_____
16. Wasp	_____	20. Wince	_____

Suggestion: Transcribe an X if the sound is correct or, if incorrect, phonetically transcribe the error. Ignore errors produced elsewhere in the word.

Comments/Notes:

Stimulability Tests for [s]

Student's Name: _____

Date: _____

Referral: _____

Imitation

   1. <u>s</u>un   _____

   2. bu<u>s</u>   _____

Best Bet Environments

End of a syllable or word

   1. ki<u>ss</u>   _____

   2. [i<u>s</u>]   _____

Before a high front vowel

   1. <u>s</u>ee   _____

   2. <u>s</u>eat   _____

After [t] and before [i]

   1. [ts<u>i</u>]   _____

   2. pi<u>zz</u>a   _____

After a [t] occurring in the same syllable

   1. beat<u>s</u>   _____

   2. [it<u>s</u>]   _____

Favorite Words

Names of family members: _____

Favorite people, heroes, and activities: _____

Phonetic Placement _____

1. Place a tongue depressor just behind the student's upper or lower front teeth, depending on which variety of [s] is being taught, and ask him or her to use the tongue tip to hold it there.

2. Next, ask the student to keep the tongue tip still while you carefully remove the tongue depressor.

3. Ask the student to breathe out, resulting in [s].

Shaping (s) from (θ) _____

1. Ask the student to place the tongue tip between the front teeth and then gently close the teeth together.

2. Ask the student to draw back the tongue tip behind the teeth. If needed, gently push the tongue tip inward with a tongue depressor.

3. Ask the student to either raise or lower the tongue tip slightly, depending on which type of [s] is being taught, and to blow air out through the mouth, resulting in [s].

Notes/Comments:

Demonstrations for [s]

Place: Alveolar

First Method

Object: None

Instructions:

1. Instruct the student, "Please stick out your tongue."
2. Once the tongue is out, for [s] with the tongue tip raised ask the student to pull the tongue back to feel the bump on the roof of the mouth behind the two front teeth. For [s] with the tongue tip down, ask the student to pull the tongue back to feel the little bump behind the two lower teeth.

Second Method

Objects: Q-tip, peanut butter or other favored food

Instructions:

1. Instruct the student, "Please open your mouth."
2. One the mouth is open, with Q-tip dab a little peanut butter or other favorite food on alveolar ridge (for tongue tip raised [s]) or behind lower front teeth (for tongue tip lowered [s]).
3. Ask the student to touch the food with the tongue tip.

Manner: Fricative

First Method

Objects: Strip of paper or a feather

Instructions:

1. Place a strip of paper, a feather, or the student's hand held in front of your mouth while you produce several long voiceless fricatives.
2. Draw attention to the "hissing" quality and continuous nature of the sounds.

Second Method

Objects: A small paper flower on end of a pencil

Instructions: Tape a small paper flower on the end of a pencil and encourage the student to move the flower in the wind.

Third Method

Objects: None

Instructions: Run your finger or the student's finger down the student's arm while making several long voiceless fricatives to demonstrate the "hissing" quality and length of fricatives.

Voicing: Voiceless

First Method

Objects: None

Instructions: Instruct the student to listen to and identify the difference between a voiceless and voiced [a].

Second Method

Objects: None

Instructions: Place the student's hands over the ears and instruct him or her to hum, which heightens the sensation of vocal cord vibration.

Third Method

Objects: None

Instructions: If the student is able to produce a voiced and voiceless fricative, ask him or her to cover the ears and make these sounds. Alternatively, ask the student to make [h] and [a].

Fourth Method

Objects: None

Instructions: You and the student place one hand on your throat and the other on the student's throat while making voiced and voiceless sounds together, telling each other when the voicing goes on and off.

Fifth Method

Objects: Pencil, small piece of paper or small paper flower

Instructions: If the student is able to produce a voiced and voiceless oral stop, attach a small piece of paper or a paper flower to the end of a tongue depressor or pencil and ask the student to "make the paper (or flower) move." The paper is more likely to move when a voiceless consonant is produced than when a voiced consonant is produced (be careful in providing instructions to the student, however, because a strongly articulated voiced oral stop will also move the flower).

Phonetic Placement and Shaping Techniques for [s]

Phonetic Placement Techniques

A key to making [s] is correct tongue tip placement. To make [s] the tongue tip is behind either the upper or lower front teeth, the upper and lower teeth are relatively close, and a narrow stream of air hisses between the tongue tip and the teeth. Once this is achieved, the hiss of air is achieved simply by breathing out, and getting the jaw relatively closed so the upper and lower teeth nearly touch is usually achieved with a few simple instructions. All the following phonetic placement techniques focus on placing the tongue tip for [s]. The first two methods are used either for [s] with the tongue tip raised or lowered, the third and fourth are for [s] with the tongue tip raised, and the fifth is for [s] with the tongue tip lowered.

First Method (tongue tip up or down) _____

This method and the following method work whether the tongue tip is up or down.

Objects: None

Instructions:

1. Ask the student to place the tongue tip behind either the upper or lower front teeth and then to pull the tongue back a little bit.
2. Close the student's teeth so the teeth barely touch.
3. Place your finger in front of the center of the student's mouth, and say "Breathe slowly over your tongue toward my finger." The sound produced by the student when breathing out approximates [s].

Second Method (tongue tip up or down) _____

Objects: Tongue depressor or Q-tip

Instructions:

1. Place a tongue depressor just behind the student's upper or lower front teeth and ask the student to use the tongue tip to hold it there.

2. Ask the student to keep the tongue still while you carefully remove the tongue depressor.
3. Ask the student to breathe out, resulting in [s].

Third Method (tongue tip up)

This method is a little more involved than the previous two. It is useful for a student who really doesn't seem to "get" the idea that the tongue tip must be raised.

Objects: Tongue depressor

Instructions:

1. Make a shelf by placing a tongue depressor against the lower edges of the student's upper teeth.
2. Next, ask the student to place the tongue on the shelf. If needed, place a tongue depressor under the student's tongue tip to bring the "elevator up" so that the tongue depressor touches the lower front teeth.
3. Ask the student to breathe out through the mouth. The resulting sound approximates [s].

Fourth Method (tongue tip up)

This somewhat involved method is for a student whose difficulty is raising the tongue and who may also experience difficulty grooving the tongue. Differing from previous methods, this one utilizes the fact that the sides of the tongue touch the inside of the teeth when making an [s]. Some children find "anchoring" the tongue sides to the teeth a helpful strategy when attempting to raise the tongue tip for [s].

Objects: Straw

Instructions:

1. Ask the student to raise his or her tongue so that the sides are firmly in contact with the inner surface of the upper back teeth. (An alternative method is to instruct the student to stick out the tongue slightly, lower the upper teeth to come into contact with the sides of the tongue, and then pull the tongue inside the mouth.)
2. Ask the student to groove the tongue slightly along the midline. (If needed, ask the student to protrude the tongue and place a clean object such as a

drinking straw along the midline of the tongue. Then ask the student to raise the sides of the tongue slightly around the straw.)

3. Carefully withdraw the straw.
4. Ask the student to place the tongue tip about a quarter of an inch behind the upper teeth and then ask the student to bring the teeth together.
5. Instruct the student to blow air along the groove of the tongue toward the lower teeth. If the student has difficulty directing the air along the tongue groove, insert a drinking straw into the student's mouth and instruct the student to blow through the straw, which often results in [s].

Fifth Method (tongue tip down)

This method works surprisingly well with some students. It can be tried for [s] with the tongue tip raised, though my clinical experience is that it is usually more effective for the tongue tip-lowered variety of [s].

Objects: None

Instructions:

1. Ask the student to brush his or her lower gums with the tongue while attempting to say [s].
2. Ask the student to stop moving the tongue and to bring the upper and lower teeth close together, but not touching.
3. Instruct the student to breathe out through the mouth, resulting in [s].

Shaping Techniques

(s) from (z)

If a student can make a [z], he or she can usually be taught to make an [s] fairly easily.

Objects: None

Instructions:

Instruct the student to say [z] and then to turn off the voice box. For some students, this is sufficient to result in [s]. (*Note:* To facilitate [z], instruct the student to turn on the voice while saying [s].)

(s) from (θ)

This method works well either for a student who lisps or one who otherwise has a well-established interdental consonant.

Objects: tongue depressor

Instructions:

1. Instruct the student to protrude the tongue between the teeth and to say [ ].
2. As the student says [θ], instruct him or her to bring the tongue back into the mouth and behind the upper or lower front teeth, depending on which variety of [s] is being facilitated. An alternative method is to ask the student to scrape the tongue tip back along the back of the front teeth. (If needed, the tip of the student's tongue can be pushed inward with a tongue depressor.)
3. Next, ask the student to either raise or lower the tongue tip slightly, depending on which type of [s] is being taught.
4. Ask the student to blow air through the mouth. The sound produced approximates [s]. (*Note:* To facilitate [z], develop from [ð].)

(s) from (ls)

These four methods help a student to convert a lateral [s] into [s].

First Method (tongue tip raised)

The following description of the useful butterfly technique is a condensed version of a Web page provided by Caroline Bowen, here: http://members.tripod .com/CarolineBowen/fsd-butterfly-procedure.htm. The technique can be applied to lateral or palatal alveolar fricatives and requires a student to be able to pronounce a correct [t] and [d].

Objects: None

Instructions:

1. Talk about the "*butterfly position*" for the tongue, or the position the tongue is in when you prolong the *i* in *pip* or the *ee* in *peep*. Point out to the student that the lateral margins of the tongue are in contact with the teeth: like a butterfly with its wings up. Older students sometimes like and are amused by the imagery of a butterfly assuming the "bracing position."
2. Draw the student's attention to the way the tongue edges (wings) press quite firmly on their teeth. You might mention that "floppy edges" or "floppy

wings" let the air out sideways, while "strong edges" or "strong wings" do not. Help the student imagine the midline of the tongue as the butterfly's body, visualizing the groove that forms along its center.

3. Tell the student the groove is there for them to "shoot" the air down, straight out in front. It is there especially to guide the air in the right direction for a super sounding *ess*. Use your hands to convey the idea of "wings up," "wings firmly tucked in against the teeth," and language such as, "a nice little groove where the butterfly's body sits," and a "straight shot" of air. Employ imagery to talk about "shooting straight" and "shooting sideways."

4. Next, model [t] and have the student imitate your production. Do the same with [t-t], then [t-t-t] and then [t-t-t-t]. If the student is producing a schwa or other vowel between the consonants, eliminate it if possible. Aim for a "pure" sounding sequence of consonants. If the student needs a vowel to get from one [t] to the next use *i* as in *pip* (ti- ti- ti-) or *ee* as in *peep* (tee-tee- tee-). Some clinicians prefer *ee* because it creates a firmer "seal" between the tongue margins and the teeth, and, potentially anyway, this discourages lateral airflow.

5. Increase the rate at which the student repeats [t-t-t-t]. Notice the subtle [s] that starts occurring between the t's. Point this out to the student in your speech and in his/her speech. The sequence is now starting to sound like [ts-ts-ts-ts].

6. The student will probably be unaware at this stage that the little "under-articulated" [s] is there. In this step, tell the student to produce the [t] and to let a little air come out at the end of the sound. Demonstrate what you mean, without actually instructing the student to produce "t and then s." Just emphasize that you want to have "air happening" after the [t]. Gradually "sharpen" the [ts] thus produced, so that it becomes obvious that there are two sounds, [t] and [s], being articulated clearly. Once it's perfect, have the student practice saying [ts] until he or she can do it very easily. It is a good idea to stay on this level for several days.

7. Now put the [ts] combination into real words. Again using the vowels *ee* as in *feet* or *i* as in *fit* to facilitate correct placement, present the student with a practice list. For example, "He eats meat, She eats candy, It eats grain," and so forth; or, "It's a boy, it's a man, it's a cow," and so forth or, "It's good, it's bad, it's tall," etc. In making up the phrases or sentences, do not include other words containing [s] or [z]. This means don't have items such as "He eats pasta" or "It's a zoo" or "It's silly." Once [ts] is established in words, practice [ts] in simple sentences that do not contain other *s*-words.

8. When the [s] the student is producing sounds clear and "adultlike," it is ready to separate from the [t]. Without mentioning the tongue too often, instruct the student to say [ts] without moving the tongue, and then add an *ess*, like this: [ts-s]. This may be difficult for the student at first, so take it slowly and quietly and give plenty of support and encouragement.

9. Next, instruct the student to make the [ts] silent, resulting in [s].

Second Method (tongue tip raised or lowered)

Objects: drinking straw

Instructions:

1. Demonstrate air flowing through a straw protruding from the side of the mouth when a lateral [s] is made and air flowing through a straw placed in the front of the mouth when a correct [s] is made.
2. Encourage the student to close the teeth and to direct the airflow through a straw placed in front of the mouth. This typically results in [s]. (*Note:* To facilitate [z], develop from lateral [z]).

Third Method (tongue tip raised or lowered)

Objects: Q-tip, picture of a small circle on a piece of paper

Instructions:

1. Instruct the student to produce a lateral [s] ([ls]).
2. Draw imaginary circles with a Q-tip where the groove should occur in the center of the tongue to indicate to the student where the air should flow during [s].
3. Next, draw a small circle on a piece of paper and hold it in front of the student's mouth at the point where air should be emitted if the air flows over the top of the tongue.
4. Instruct the student to direct the air through the circle while saying [s]. An alternative method is to instruct the student to use the fingers instead of paper. If the student's fingers are used, the sensation of air is felt more keenly if the fingers are wet. (*Note:* To facilitate [z], develop from lateral [z].)

Fourth Method (tongue tip raised or lowered)

Objects: None

Instructions:

1. Ask the student to gently bite the sides of the tongue, drop the tongue tip, and put it behind the front teeth.
2. Ask the student to smile and blow air out the front of the mouth, resulting in [s].

(s) from (t)

These methods rely on the fact that [t] and [s] are made in the same place of production. It is extremely helpful for the many students who have a well-established [t]. A limitation on its utility is that it requires the student to follow a number of steps, which some students find challenging.

First Method

Objects: None

Instructions:

1. Instruct the student to say [t] in *tea* with strong aspiration. If said quickly and forcefully, [tsi] results. An alternative to this procedure is to ask the student to say [tsi] instead of *tea*.
2. Instruct the student to say [tsi] without the vowel, resulting in [ts].
3. Ask the student to prolong the [s] portion of [ts], resulting in *tsss*.
4. Ask the student to make [t] silent, resulting in [s].

Second Method

Objects: None

Instructions:

1. Ask the student to open the mouth and to put the tongue in position for [t].
2. Instruct the student to lower the tongue slightly and to send the air over the tongue.
3. Place the student's finger in front of the mouth to feel the emission of air, which typically results in [s].

Third Method

This is a clever variation of the [s] from [t] method that was developed by Gillian Fleming of Dunedin, New Zealand, who kindly consented to let it be placed in this book. It works especially well for establishing [s] at the end of words. Gillian writes, "I feel that by the time a child reaches school age, he/she is very aware of the [s] sound. People have been trying to correct it for ages, saying things like, 'Put your tongue in' or 'It's not [θ], it's [s]' and other unhelp-

ful comments. The child is programmed to use their lateral sound or their lisp as soon as they see or think about [s]. So, when they first present for therapy, I tell them we are not going to work on [s]—we are going to work on making good clear [t] sounds."

Objects: None

Instructions:

1. Instruct the student to make the tongue tip on the ridge behind the top teeth, resulting in a series of short [t] sounds (t—t—t—t—t).
2. Next, instruct the student to make [t] a little longer (ttt ttt ttt).
3. Next, make [t] a little longer still (tttttt—tttttttt—tttttt).
4. Lastly, put the long tttttt on the end of a word (catttt—big catttt—fluffy cattttt—etc.), resulting in word final [ts].
5. Once clear [s] is established, practice final [ts] in other words (*bats*, *boats*, *kites*, etc.)
6. When the clinician feels the time is right, point out that the student is now making a correct [s] sound.

(s) from (ʃ)

As this method attests, sometimes the only thing that is needed to succeed is a good smile. Retracting the lips to smile pulls the tongue forward into an [s].

Objects: None

Instructions:

1. Ask the student to say [ʃ].
2. Ask the student to retract the lips into a smile. Often, this moves the tongue forward slightly into the position for [s]. If needed, however, ask the student to move the tongue slightly forward, resulting in [s]. (*Note:* To facilitate [z], develop from [voiced ʃ] or instruct the student to turn on the voice box.)

(s) from (f)

This method, like the one above, converts one fricative into another. The difference is that it approaches [s] from an anterior position rather than a posterior one. I have found it a little less successful than the previous method.

Objects: None

Instructions:

1. Ask the student to lift the tongue tip slowly while making a prolonged [f].
2. Ask the student to bring the front teeth close together but not quite touching. If needed, gently pull out the student's lower lip slightly.
3. Ask the student to smile while making the sound, which often results in [s]. (*Note:* To facilitate [z], develop from [v] or use [s] and instruct the student to turn on his or her voice box.)

(s) from (i)

Admittedly, this and the method that follows are a somewhat far stretch. This method relies on the similarity in the place of production of [i] and [s], and the following method relies on similarity in the frication created by [s] and [h]. Neither would be my first choice for a method to remediate [s], but each has a place in the clinical repertoire.

Objects: None

Instructions:

1. Instruct the student to say [i].
2. Ask the student to turn off the voice and gradually close the teeth until [s] results (*Note:* To facilitate [z], instruct the student to keep the voice box on.)

(s) from (h)

Objects: None

Instructions:

1. Ask the student to gradually close the teeth while saying [h].
2. Ask the student to raise the tongue tip gradually while producing a prolonged [h] until the resulting sound is [s]. (*Note:* To facilitate [z], instruct the student to turn on the voice.)

Shell for Speech Exercises

Student's Name: _____

Date: _____

Treatment Sound: _____

Word List: Student Responses:

                                          1. _____

                                          2. _____

                                          3. _____

                                          4. _____

                                          5. _____

                                          6. _____

                                          7. _____

                                          8. _____

                                          9. _____

                                        10. _____

Total Correct: _____ / _____

Comments:

Imitation

Student's Name: _____

Date: _____

Treatment Sound: _____

Goal: Have the student repeat the word after you.

Instructions to Student: "You are going to hear a word with our sound. Please say it after me. Here's an example. I say *sat*, and then you say *sat*."

Word List: **Student Responses:**

Sat   1. _____

Salmon   2. _____

Sail   3. _____

Salad   4. _____

Sailboat   5. _____

Socks   6. _____

Soap   7. _____

Sew   8. _____

Sun   9. _____

Sally   10. _____

Total Correct: _____/_____

Comments:

Minimal Pairs

Student's Name: _____

Date: _____

Treatment Sound: _____

Goal: Have the student first say the word with the treatment sound, then say the rhyming word, and then say the word with the treatment sound.

Instructions to Student: "You are going to hear a word that begins with our sound. Please say the word, then replace our sound with another sound to make the word have a different meaning, and then say the word with our sound again. Here's an example. I say *seal*. You say *seal*, then change [s] to [w] to make *wheel*, and then say *seal* again. Like this: *Seal. Wheel. Seal.*"

Word List:		Student Responses:
Sink	think	1. _____
Ceiling	peeling	2. _____
Sip	whip	3. _____
Soak	poke	4. _____
Sea	me	5. _____
Son	fun	6. _____
Sad	mad	7. _____
Sack	back	8. _____
Sun	fun	9. _____
Sick	tick	10. _____

Total Correct: _____ / _____

Comments:

Deletion

Student's Name: _____

Date: _____

Treatment Sound: _____

Goal: Have the student first say the word with the treatment sound, then without the treatment sound, and then with the treatment sound.

Instructions to Student: "You are going to hear a word with our sound. Please say the word, and then say it with our sound deleted, and then say it with our sound included. Here's an example. I say *red*. You say *red*, then *Ed*, then *red*. Like this: *Red. Ed. Red.*"

Word List:		Student Responses:
Sat	at	1. _____
Sail	ale, ail	2. _____
Sew	O, oh	3. _____
Sally	alley	4. _____
Silk	ilk	5. _____
Sea gull	eagle	6. _____
Sick	ick	7. _____
Sole	ole	8. _____
Sink	ink	9. _____
Sea	E	10. _____

Total Correct: _____ / _____

Comments:

Self-Correction

Student's Name: _____

Date: _____

Treatment Sound: _____

Goal: Have the student say the word three times, self-correcting if errors in the treatment sound occur.

Instructions to Student: "You are going to hear a word with our sound. Please say the word three times, listening to how you say our sound and changing it to make it correctly if you say it incorrectly. Here's an example. I say *cheese*, and then you say *cheese* three times, listening to how you say our sound and changing it to make it correctly if you say it incorrectly. Like this: *Cheese. Cheese. Cheese.*"

Word List:	Student Responses:
Sat	1. _____
Salmon	2. _____
Sail	3. _____
Salad	4. _____
Sailboat	5. _____
Socks	6. _____
Soap	7. _____
Sew	8. _____
Sun	9. _____
Sally	10. _____

Total Correct: _____ / _____

Comments:

Old Way/New Way

Student's Name: _____

Date: _____

Treatment Sound: _____

Goal: Have the student say the word the new way, the old way, and then the new way again.

Instructions to Student: "You are going to hear a word with our sound. Please say the word, then say it the old way you used to say our sound, and then say it the new way you say our sound. Here's an example. I say *thin*. You say *thin*, then **in*, and then *thin*. Like this: *Thin. *in. Thin.*"

Note: Replace * with the way the student used to say the sound.

Word List:	Student Responses:
Sat	1. _____
Salmon	2. _____
Sail	3. _____
Salad	4. _____
Sailboat	5. _____
Socks	6. _____
Soap	7. _____
Sew	8. _____
Sun	9. _____
Sally	10. _____

Total Correct: _____/_____

Comments:

Similar Sound

Student's Name: _____

Date: _____

Treatment Sound: _____

Goal: Have the student first say the word with the treatment sound, then with the most similar sound the student can make, and then with the treatment sound again.

Instructions to Student: "You are going to hear a word with our sound. Please say the word, then replace our sound with _____*, and then say the word with our sound. Here's an example. I say *sun*. You say *sun*, then **un*, and then *sun* again. Like this: *Sun. *un. Sun.*"

Note: Replace * with a sound the student can pronounce that is phonetically similar to the treatment sound.

Word List: **Student Responses:**

Sat   1. _____

Salmon   2. _____

Sail   3. _____

Salad   4. _____

Sailboat   5. _____

Socks   6. _____

Soap   7. _____

Sew   8. _____

Sun   9. _____

Sally   10. _____

Total Correct: _____ / _____

Comments:

Complete Word List for [s]

Beginning of Words

Single Consonants	*Deletions*	*Minimal Pairs*
Sat	at	bat, mat, hat, cat, rat, pat
Salmon		
Sail	ale, ail	tail, pail, nail, veil, rail, whale, mail, jail
Salad		ballad
Sailboat		
Socks		fox, rocks, box
Soap		rope
Sew	O, oh	toe, row, hoe, no, bow, mow, go
Sun		fun, run, one, bun, gun
Sally	alley	tally
Silk	ilk	
Sea gull	eagle	
Sick	ick	tick, thick, kick, pick, lick, wick
Sole	ole	mole, goal, hole
Saber		
Sink	ink	think, pink, rink, wink
Surgeon		
Sea	E	me, bee, key, knee, pea
Cellar		teller
Sioux	oo	dew, coo
Saddle	addle	paddle
Surfboard		
Sailboat		
Son		fun, run, bun, gun, one
Sidewalk		
Sand	and	band, fanned, tanned, hand
Surfer		
Sunrise		
Sad	add	mad, bad, dad
Sundae		fun day
Sydney		kidney
Sunday		fun day
Sunburn		
Susan		
Cycle		Michael

Single Consonants	Deletions	Minimal Pairs
Circle		
Sit	it	hit, mit, kit, knit, bit
Soldier		
Sam	am	ham, lamb
Salesclerk		
Six		wicks, mix
Seaweed		
Suit		cute, hoot, boot
Cindy	Indy	windy
Soar	or, oar	four, more, tore, bore, core
Ceiling		peeling, reeling, kneeling
Sub		hub, cub
Sunlight		
Saint	ain't	paint, faint
Subway		
Seal	eel	Neil, heel
Cement		
Sour	hour	tower, shower, cower
Sunny		honey, money, funny, bunny
Suck	uck	buck, luck, shuck, muck
City		kitty, witty
Soup		loop, poop
Salt	ought	malt
Sign		nine, fine, shine
Sandal		handle
Sid	id	hid, kid, bid, lid
Song		thong, long
Sank		rank, lank, bank
Suds		duds, cuds
Soak	oak	poke, choke, yolk, joke, woke
Serve		Merv, curve
Sound		round, pound
Sue	ooh	boo, who, due
Soot		foot
Sing		wing, thing, king, ring
Sip		whip, rip, lip, hip, dip
Cell	L	fell, dell, Mel
Sack		back, rack, hack, pack, tack
Surf		turf
Soil	oil	boil, coil
Sock		lock, mock

Consonant Clusters   *Deletions*

(sp)

Spot	pot
Spell	
Spicy	
Spout	pout
Spanish	
Space	pace
Spill	pill
Spit	pit
Spokes	pokes
Spider	
Sponge	
Spear	peer
Spark	park
Spank	
Spoon	
Spare ribs	
Spin	pin
Spy	pie
Spade	paid
Spooky	Pooky
Spy	pie
Spaceship	
Spike	pike
Spirit	
Speak	peak
Special	
Spear	peer
Speed	peed

(st)

Stop	top
Sting	ting
Stoplight	
Stink	
Story	Tory
Stack	tack
Stork	torque
Stagecoach	
Steak	take

Consonant Clusters	Deletions
Stick	tick
Storm	
Stairs	tears
Stone Age	
Stalk	talk
Stool	tool
Stallion	
Staff	
Steam	team
Steal	teal
Starfish	
Stamp	
Stale	tale, tail
Stock car	
Stand	
Stub	tub
Star	tar
Stew	two
Staff	
Stag	
Stake	take
Standard	
Statue	
Steady	Teddy

(sk)

School	cool
Ski	key, C
Skin	kin
Scale	kale
Skinny	
Skirt	Kurt
Skier	
Scarf	
School bus	cool bus
Scar	car
Skate	Kate
Scotland	
Skunk	
Skip	Kip
Sky	

Consonant Clusters	Deletions
Skillful	
Skirt	Kurt
Sketch	
Skew	Q
Skim	Kim
Skull	cull
Skid	kid
Skill	kill

(sf)

Sphinx	finks
Sphere	fear
Sphincter	

(sl)

Slip	lip
Sleigh	lay
Slide	lied
Sleep	leap
Sled dog	
Slug	lug
Sling	
Sled	led
Slimy	limey
Sleepy	
Sleeve	leave
Slippers	
Sliver	liver
Slime	lime
Sloth	
Slab	lab
Slang	
Slick	lick
Slump	lump
Slow	low
Slash	lash
Slink	link
Slate	late
Slave	
Slop	

Consonant Clusters	Deletions
Slay	lay
Sleek	leak
Sliver	liver

(sw)

Swing	wing
Swimmer	
Sweater	wetter
Sweatshirt	
Sweet tooth	
Sweat	wet
Swiss	
Sweet	wheat
Switch	witch
Swamp	
Swim	whim
Swan	wan
Swelter	welter
Swerve	
Swear	wear
Sweden	
Swat	watt
Sweep	weep
Sway	way
Swap	
Swallow	wallow
Swarm	warm
Swift	wift

(sm)

Small	mall
Smell	Mel
Smile	mile
Smelly	
Smog	
Smoke	
Smack	Mack
Smoky	
Smooth	
Smallest	

Consonant Clusters	Deletions
Smock	mock
Smart	mart
Smoky	
Smash	mash
Smother	mother
Smudge	
Smite	mite

(sn)

Snack	knack
Snail	nail
Snout	
Snorkel	
Snap	nap
Snake bite	
Snow	no, know
Snarl	gnarl
Snack bar	
Snow bank	no bank
Snow White	no white
Sneakers	
Snoopy	
Snake	
Sneeze	knees
Snore	nor
Sneer	near
Snug	
Sniff	
Snippy	nippy
Sniffle	
Snub	nub
Sneak	
Snatch	
Snob	knob
Snort	

(spr)

Spring	
Spray	pray
Sprite (soda)	

Consonant Clusters	Deletions
Sprinkle	
Spry	pry
Spray gun	
Spruce	
Sprint	print
Sprinkles	
Springboard	
Sprinkling	
Springtime	
Sprain	
Spread	
Sprig	prig
Spree	
Spruce	
Sprout	

(str)

Struck	truck
Strum	
Strike out	
Strong	
Stroller	troller
Street	treat
Stranger	
Straw	
Stronghold	
Stripe	tripe
String	
Strike zone	
Streetcar	
Stream	
Strap	trap
Strike	trike
Stretcher	
Strict	tricked
Stroke	
Struggle	
Strum	
Strut	

Consonant Clusters   *Deletions*

(skr)

Screen	
Scribble	
Scream	cream
Scratch	
Scrapper	
Scrooge	
Screenplay	
Scrub	
Screw	crew
Screen	
Script	crypt
Scramble	
Scribe	
Scrap	crap
Scroll	
Scrimp	crimp
Scrabble	
Screech	

(skw)

Square	
Squash	
Squeal	keel
Squeak	
Squad	quad
Squirt	
Squaw	
Squalid	
Squash	
Squirm	
Squeeze	
Squall	
Squint	
Squadron	

(spl)

Splashdown
Splinter

Consonant Clusters   Deletions

Split
Splash
Splint
Spleen
Splat
Splice
Splurge

(s) + Stops (p t k)   Deletions

Sting	ting
Spicy	
Skirt	Kurt
Steak	take
Spanish	
Staff	
Skull	cull
Steady	Teddy
Skinny	
Spill	pill
Spider	
Skirt	Kurt
Sponge	
Sketch	
Skew	Q
Skim	Kim
Spear	peer
Scotland	
Spark	park
Skid	kid
Spareribs	
Steal	teal
Spin	pin
Staff	
Spy	pie
Skill	kill
Spade	paid
Stoplight	top light
Spooky	Pooky
Spy	lie
Stone Age	

(s) + Stops (p t k)   Deletions

Stallion	
Starfish	
Spaceship	
Stop	top
Spot	pot
Stag	
Stake	take
Spit	pit
Story	Tory
Spirit	
Stack	tack
Spoon	
Stork	
Stagecoach	
Space	pace
Stick	tick
Storm	
Stairs	tears
Spank	
Stalk	talk
Sky	
Stool	tool
Special	
Skip	Kip
Stamp	
Spike	pike
Speed	peed
Stock car	
Spokes	pokes
Stand	
Stub	tub
Star	tar
Stew	two
School	cool
Standard	
Ski	key
Speak	peak
Skin	kin
Spout	pout
Scale	kale
Spell	
Skier	

(s) + Stops (p t k)   Deletions

Scarf	
Spear	peer
School bus	cool bus
Stink	
Scar	car
Steam	team
Skate	Kate
Statue	
Skunk	
Stale	tale, tail

(s) + Nasals (m n)   Deletions

Small	mall
Snarl	gnarl
Sneeze	knees
Smell	
Snail	nail
Smock	mock
Sneer	near
Snort	
Smile	mile
Snoopy	
Smog	
Snow White	no white
Smoke	
Snug	
Snob	knob
Smart	mart
Smite	mite
Snack bar	
Smooth	
Snoopy	
Smoky	
Smudge	
Snake	
Smallest	
Snack	knack
Snub	nub
Sneak	
Smother	mother

(s) + Nasals (m n)   Deletions

Snout	
Smack	Mack
Snorkel	
Snap	nap
Smash	mash
Snake bite	
Smelly	
Snow	no, know
Smoky	
Sniff	
Snippy	nippy
Sniffle	
Snatch	
Snow bank	no bank
Sneakers	
Snore	nor

(s) + Two Consonants   Deletions

Squeal	keel
Strike	trike
Stretcher	
Screw	crew
Spread	
Squeak	
Spray	pray
Squalid	
Strap	trap
Screen	
Screech	
Sprinkle	
Sprinkles	
Scrimp	crimp
Scrabble	
Street	treat
Squash	
Squirm	
Sprinkling	
Struck	truck
Script	crypt
Scramble	

(s) + Two Consonants   Deletions

Scribe	
Sprain	
Squint	
Squadron	
Strum	
Squall	
Splash	
Strike out	
Squeeze	
Springtime	
Scrap	crap
Scroll	
Strong	
Spray gun	
Strict	tricked
Stroke	
Spruce	
Stroller	
Splint	
Scream	cream
Stranger	
Sprig	prig
Straw	
Sprint	print
Stronghold	
Squad	quad
Spree	
Stripe	tripe
Split	
String	
Strike zone	
Squash	
Struggle	
Strum	
Scrooge	
Streetcar	
Square	
Scrapper	
Splurge	
Squirt	
Stream	
Splashdown	

(s) + Two Consonants   **Deletions**

Spring
Sprite (soda)
Strut
Splinter
Screen
Spruce
Sprout
Scribble
Splat
Splice
Scratch
Screenplay
Scrub
Spleen
Squeak
Springboard
Squaw

Medial

Single Consonants

Icy	Racer	Jason
Dress up	Russell	Glasses
Muscle	Castle	Lucy
Acid	Fossil	Mossy
Messy	Grassy	Posse
Icing	Brussels	Peso
Possum	Bossy	Kissing
Bison	Tracy	Bessie
Lassie	Racing	Casey
Faucet	Listen	Tracing
Dissect	Tucson	

Consonant Clusters

Hopscotch	Shoe store	Einstein
Ice skate	Explore	Casper
Crystal	Pretzel	Hairspray
Oscar	Eskimo	Bus stop
Costume	Shakespeare	Explode
Expressway	Dog sled	Pizza
Diskette	Cub Scout	Asleep
Ski slope	Basking	Baseman
Basement	Shoestring	Whisker
Whisper	Postman	Hot spring
Sixty	Locksmith	Houston
Chop sticks	Escape	Casket
Teaspoon	Betsy	Bracelet

All Environments

Shakespeare	Dissect	Costume
Icy	Asleep	Tucson
Dress up	Racer	Diskette
Sixty	Postman	Ski slope
Dog sled	Russell	Basement
Muscle	Castle	Whisker
Teaspoon	Betsy	Jason
Explore	Hairspray	Pizza
Acid	Fossil	Glasses
Basking	Escape	Hopscotch
Messy	Grassy	Lucy
Cub Scout	Casper	Mossy
Pretzel	Bracelet	Ice skate
Icing	Brussels	Posse
Shoe store	Einstein	Houston
Possum	Locksmith	Baseman
Chop sticks	Bossy	Peso
Oscar	Whisper	Kissing
Bison	Expressway	Crystal
Hot springs	Shoestring	Bessie
Lassie	Tracy	Bus stop
Eskimo	Explode	Casey
Faucet	Racing	Tracing
Casket	Listen	

End of Words

Single Consonants	*Deletions*
Toss	
White house	
Dice	die
Goose	goo
Moose	moo
Courthouse	
Ice	eye, I
Noose	new
Nervous	
Famous	
Trace	tray
Gas	
Red Cross	
Race	ray
Lighthouse	
Glass	
Fireplace	
Mace	May
Janis	
Greece	
Kansas	
Bruce	brew
Porpoise	
Press	
Grass	
Police	
Gross	grow
Palace	
Grease	
Air base	
Lewis	Louie
Cross	
Mattress	
Paris	
Pass	
Geese	Gee
Necklace	
Carlos	Carlo
Rice	rye

Single Consonants   Deletions

Dress
Alice   alley
Blouse
Yes
Mouse   Mao
Bus
Briefcase
Chris
Kiss
Congress
Class
Vase
Face   Fay, fey
Bernice
Ace   A
Hiss
Horse
Mice   my
Bus
Boss
Moss

Consonant Clusters   Deletions

(sp)

Wasp
Lisp   lip
Grasp
Crisp
Gasp   gap

(st)

Waist   wait
Chest   Chet
Frost   fraught
Signpost
Fast   fat
Midwest
Crust

Consonant Clusters	**Deletions**
Rust	rut
Artist	
Post	
Fist	fit
Breakfast	
Mist	mitt
August	
Feast	feet
Toast	tote
Twist	twit
Chemist	
Most	moat
Nest	net
Forest	
Gust	gut
Signpost	
Toothpaste	
West	wet
Typist	
Vest	vet
Conquest	
Priest	
August	
Gymnast	
Ghost	goat
Wrist	writ
Last	
Slowest	
Key West	
Lost	
East	eat

(sk)

Desk	deck
Mask	Mack
Disk	Dick
Corn husk	
Tusk	tuck
Mollusk	
Gas mask	
Husk	Huck

Consonant Clusters	Deletions
Ask	
School desk	
Face mask	
Whisk	wick
Task	tack
Mosque	mock

(sl)

Missile
Axle
Fossil
Muscle
Wrestle

(ls)

Convulse	
Pulse	Paul

(ns)

Fence	fen
Dance	Dan
Defense	
Florence	
Wince	win
Immense	
France	Fran
Balance	
Science	
Pounce	
Tense	ten
Prince	
Bounce	
License	
Rinse	
Lance	
Entrance	

Consonant Clusters	Deletions
(rs)	
Force	four
Divorce	
Pierce	peer
Golf course	
Fierce	fear
Hoarse	whore
Horse	whore
Air Force	
Sawhorse	
(ks)	
Ax	
Alex	
Fox	
Smallpox	
Comics	comic
Larynx	
Phoenix	
Mailbox	
Box	Bach
Tax	tack
(s) + Consonant	
Fast	fat
Wasp	
Waist	wait
Mosque	mock
Chest	Chet
Frost	fraught
Signpost	
Midwest	
Crust	
Lisp	lip
Rust	rut
Artist	
Gasp	gap
Fist	fit
Crisp	

Consonant Clusters	Deletions
Breakfast	
Mist	mitt
School desk	
August	
Feast	feet
Facemask	
Husk	Huck
Toast	tote
Twist	twit
Mollusk	
Chemist	
Most	moat
Gas mask	
Nest	net
Forest	
Wrestle	
Gust	gut
Signpost	
Toothpaste	
West	wet
Corn husk	
Typist	
Fossil	
Tusk	tuck
Frost	fraught
Vest	vet
Conquest	
Priest	
Muscle	
Gymnast	
Wrist	writ
Last	
Grasp	
Slowest	
Key West	
East	eat
Desk	deck
Post	
Mask	Mack
Ghost	goat
Disk	Dick
August	

Consonant Clusters	**Deletions**
Axle	
Ask	
Whisk	wick
Lost	
Task	tack
Missile	

Consonant + (s)

Convulse	
Rinse	
Fence	fen
Comics	comic
Larynx	
Florence	
Fierce	fear
Wince	win
Box	
Immense	
Air Force	
Dance	Dan
Horse	whore
Sawhorse	
France	Fran
Ax	
Balance	
Fox	
Smallpox	
Science	
Force	four
Pounce	
Hoarse	whore
Tense	ten
Defense	
Prince	
Phoenix	
Bounce	
Pulse	Paul
License	
Prince	
Alex	
Lance	

Consonant Clusters

Entrance
Divorce
Tax
Pierce
Golf course
Mailbox

Deletions

tack
peer

Plural Markers

Bucks
Cats
Tops
Punks
Picks
Spots
Pops
Shops
Tips
Carts
Skunks
Sharks
Pops
Droughts
Types
Spouts
Embarks
Plops
Sinks
Shouts

Deletions

buck
cat
top
punk
pick
spot
pop
shop
tip
cart
skunk
shark
pop
drought
type
spout
embark
plop
sink
shout

Themes for (s)

Themes

Snack Time
Let's Bake
Field and Forest
Horseback Riding
At the Beach
People to See
Places to Go

The Body
Speech
Bath time
Clothes to Wear
Medieval Fun
Bus Ride Around Town

Snack Time	Deletions	Minimal Pairs
Messy		
Toast	tote	
Swallow	wallow	
Spare ribs		
Soup		loop, poop
Salt	ought	malt
Sip		whip, rip, lip, hip, dip
Rice	rye	mice, lice
Salad		ballad
Sundae		fun day
Steak	take	
Sub		hub, cub
Sour	hour	tower, shower, cower
Icy		
Sprout		
Icing		
Squirm		
Sprouts	sprout	
Squeeze		
Squash		
Skim		Kim
Splurge		
Spread		
Spicy		
Spree		
Stew	two	
Sprinkle		wrinkle
Snack bar		
Snack	knack	
Smell	Mel	
Sweet	wheat	
Sprinkles		
Chopsticks		
Pizza	pita	
Crust		
Crisp		
Frosting		

Let's Bake	Deletions	Minimal Pairs
Snack	knack	
Icing		
Grease		
Feast	feet	
Crust		
Swallow		wallow
Crisp		
Frost	fraught	
Snack	knack	
Smell	Mel	
Sweet	wheat	
Sprinkles		
Whisk	wick	
Teaspoon		
Frosting		
Spoon		
Skim		Kim
Splurge		
Spread		

Field and Forest	Deletions	Minimal Pairs
Fox		
Fence	fen	
Corn husk		
Tusk	tuck	
Sprig		prig
Spruce		
Husk	Huck	
Sliver		liver
Ax		
Salmon		
Sun		fun, run, one, bun, gun
Mouse	Mao	
Saddle	addle	
Sleek		leak
Swerve		
Swan		wan
Swallow		wallow
Sailboat		
Sand	and	band, fanned, tanned, hand

Field and Forest	Deletions	Minimal Pairs
Sunrise		
Swarm		warm
Swift		wift
Sunlight		
Sunny		honey, money, funny, bunny
Soil	oil	boil, coil
Possum		
Stag		
Moose	moo	
Bison		
Grassy		
Skunk		
Skip	Kip	
Mossy		
Moss		
Stork		
Sky		
Slug	lug	
Stallion		
Stick	tick	
Storm		
Horse	whore	
Mice	my	
Grass		
Goose	goo	
Geese	gee	
Stream		
Splash		
Cycle		Michael
Forest		

Horseback Riding	Deletions	Minimal Pairs
Fence	fen	
Sun		fun, run, one, bun, gun
Saddle	addle	
Sunlight		
Sunny		honey, money, funny, bunny
Grassy		
Swift		wift
Stallion		

Storm		
Sleek		leak
Swerve		
Swelter		welter
Horse	whore	
Grass		
Stream		
Splash		
Forest		

At the Beach	*Deletions*	*Minimal Pairs*
Mollusk		
Salmon		
Sail	ale, ail	tail, pail, nail, veil, rail, whale, mail, jail
Sailboat		
Sun		fun, run, one, bun, gun
Sea gull	eagle	
Sole	ole	mole, goal, coal
Sea	E	pea, me, key
Surfboard		
Sailboat		
Sand	and	band, fanned, tanned, hand
Sunburn		
Surfer		
Sunrise		
Squall		
Sharks	shark	
Seaweed		
Sunlight		
Seal	eel	Neil, heel
Sunny		honey, money, funny, bunny
Sandal		handle
Surf		turf
Lighthouse		
Porpoise		
Sky		
Stallion		
Stick	tick	
Storm		
Starfish		kitty, witty
Splash		

People to See	Deletions	Minimal Pairs
Alex		
Lance		
Sally	alley	tally
Sioux	oo	dew, coo
Lucy	Louie	
Susan		
Russell		
Sam	am	Pam, ram, lamb
Cindy	Indy	windy
Sid	id	hid, kid, bid, Sid
Sue	ooh	boo, who, due
Lassie		
Tracy		
Jason		
Bessie		
Casey		
Janis		
Bruce	brew	
Lewis		
Carlos	Carlo	
Alice		
Chris		
Smoky		
Snow White	no white	
Oscar		
Shakespeare		
Betsy	Betty	
Einstein		
Casper		
Snoopy		

Places to Go	Deletions	Minimal Pairs
Phoenix		
France	Fran	
Florence		
Sphinx		
Sweden		
Key West		
Sydney		kidney
Tucson		

Places to Go	Deletions	Minimal Pairs
Brussels		
White House		
Greece		
Kansas		
Scotland		
Houston		

The Body	Deletions	Minimal Pairs
Larynx		
Smallpox		
Skin	kin	
Smile	mile	
Sniffle		
Splint		
Spleen		
Sprain		
Stretcher		
Stroke		
Skull		cull
Sneeze	knees	
Snore	nor	
Gasp	gap	
Lisp	lip	
Waist	wait	
Chest	Chet	
Wrist	writ	
Muscle		
Pulse	Paul	
Fist	fit	
Sick	ick	tick, thick, kick, pick, lick, wick
Snort		
Speak		peak
Squint		
Sniff		
Slump		lump

Speech	**Deletions**	**Minimal Pairs**
Slang		
Speak		peak
Lisp	lip	
Smile	mile	
Larynx		
Swear		wear

Bath Time	**Deletions**	**Minimal Pairs**
Splash		
Steam	team	
Sting	ting	
Sponge		
Spout	pout	
Spill	pill	
Face	ace	Fay, fey
Faucet		
Sing		wing, thing, king, ring
Suds		duds, cuds
Soak	oak	poke, choke, yolk, joke, woke
Soap		rope, pope
Sink	ink	think, pink, rink, wink

Clothes to Wear	**Deletions**	**Minimal Pairs**
Socks		fox, rocks, box
Sew	ooh	toe, row, hoe, no, bow, mow, go
Suit		cute, hoot, boot
Sock		lock, mock
Sneakers		
Slip	lip	
Skirt	Kurt	
Dress up		
Glasses		
Necklace		
Strap		trap
Dress		
Blouse		
Scarf		

Clothes to Wear	Deletions	Minimal Pairs
Sleeve	leave	
Slippers		
Strap	trap	
Costume		
Silk	ilk	
Shoestring		
Bracelet		
Vest	vet	

Medieval Fun	Deletions	Minimal Pairs
Saber		
Soldier		
Spell		
Story	Tory	
Saint	ain't	paint, faint
Cellar		teller
Sad	add	mad, bad, dad
Cell	L	fell, dell, Mel
Sack		back, rack, hack, pack, tack
Casket		
Sneak		
Locksmith		
Slave		
Squalid		
Stake		take
Slay		lay
Escape		
Crystal		
Straw		
Swing	wing	
Scar	car	
Staff		
Struggle		
Staff		
Spike		pike
Spirit		
Splat		
Strike		trike
Spear		peer
Speed		peed

Medieval Fun	*Deletions*	*Minimal Pairs*
Swat		watt
Scribe		
Scroll		
Sneer		near
Slash		lash
Slink		link
Stairs	tears	
Spy	pie	
Spade	paid	
Spooky	Pooky	
Spy	lie	
Spider		
Spear	peer	
Castle		
Fireplace		
Mace	May	
Palace		
Cross		
Spark	park	
Stalk	talk	
Swamp		
Smoke		
Stronghold		
Squad	quad	
Conquest		
Priest		
Nest	net	
Forest		
Mist	mitt	
Gust	gut	
Ghost	goat	
Lost		
Mask	Mack	
Wrestle		
Defense		
Prince		
Entrance		
Force	four	
Pierce	peer	
Fierce	fear	
Horse	whore	
Feast	feet	

Bus Ride Around Town	Deletions	Minimal Pairs
Sat	at	bat, mat, hat, cat, rat, pat
Sit	it	hit, mit, kit, knit, bit
Subway		
City		witty, kitty
Cement		
Sign		nine, fine, shine
Sidewalk		
Salesclerk		
Postman		
Stroller		
Street	treat	
Stand		
Stop	top	
Pass		
Courthouse		
Police		
Bus		
Briefcase		
Stoplight	top light	
School bus	cool bus	
Switch	witch	
Shoe store		
Bus stop		

Chapter Five

[z]

Definition

[z] is made in either of two ways. As with [s], some people produce [z] with the tongue tip up behind the upper front teeth, others say it with the tongue tip down behind the lower front teeth. Neither one is the "right way." Follow the student's lead in deciding which way to teach [z]. If the student appears to find it easier to say [z] with the tongue tip up, teach the sounds that way; if the student appears to find it easier to say [z] with the tongue tip down, teach the sound that way. For both varieties of [z], the airstream is continuous and the vocal folds are together. The technical definition of [z] is voiced alveolar fricative.

Acquisition

50% of children acquire [s] by 4;0 and 75% of children acquire [s] by 6;0.

Relative Frequency

[z] is ranked 5th in relative frequency compared to the other late-acquired consonants. It ranks 15th in relative frequency compared to all other English consonants, and its percentage of occurrence compared to all English consonants is 3.0%.

Errors

[z] is affected by many of the same errors as [s]—Lisping, Bladed productions, and Lateralizing are all common errors for [z]. Additionally, at the end of words [z] may be produced with little or no voicing, resulting in an [s]-like sound.

Key Environments

End of a syllable or word, as in *fizz*
Before a high front vowel, as in *zip*
After [d] and before [i], as in *[dzi]*
After a [d] occurring in the same syllable, as in **beads**

Possible Metaphors

Select metaphors based on the aspect of speech that is the focus of therapy.

Tongue placement:	Tongue tip sound,
	Bmp sound (tongue tip up)
	Little hill sound (tongue tip up)
	Lower teeth sound (tongue tip down)
Fricative:	Snake sound
	Long sound
	Hissing sound
Voicing:	Motor on
	Buzzing sound
	Voice box on sound

Touch Cue

Finger on the corner of the mouth (finger up for tongue tip raised sound or finger down for tongue tip down sound).

Instruction:

Place the student's finger in the corner of the lips, and remind the student to keep upper and lower teeth close together.

Initial Screening Test for [z]

Student's Name: _____

Date: _____

Referral: _____

Instructions: Say to the student, "I'm going to say some words. Please say the words after me."
Example: "Dog. Now you say it."

Word	Student*
Beginning	
1. Zen	_____
2. Zone	_____
3. Zombie	_____
Medial	
4. Daisy	_____
5. Rosa	_____
6. Moses	_____
Final	
7. Nose	_____
8. Buzz	_____
9. Hose	_____

*Suggestion: Transcribe an X if the sound is correct or, if incorrect, phonetically transcribe the error. Ignore errors produced elsewhere in the word.

Comments/Notes:

Stimulability Tests for [z]

Student's Name: _____

Date: _____

Referral: _____

Imitation

  1. zoo   _____

  2. buzz   _____

Best Bet Environments

End of a syllable or word

  1. fizz   _____

  2. [iz]   _____

Before a high front vowel

  1. zip   _____

  2. zero   _____

After [d] and before [i]

  1. [dzi]   _____

After a [d] occurring in the same syllable

  1. beads   _____

  2. ads   _____

Favorite Words

Names of family members: _____

Favorite people, heroes, and activities: _____

Phonetic Placement   _____

1. Place a tongue depressor just behind the student's upper or lower front teeth, depending on which variety of /z/ is being taught, and ask him or her to use the tongue tip to hold it there.

2. Next, ask the student to keep the tongue tip still while you carefully remove the tongue depressor.

3. Ask the student to breathe out, resulting in [s].

4. Ask student to turn voice box on, resulting in [z].

Shaping (z) from (s) ⸺⸺⸺

Instruct the student to say [s] and then to turn on the voice box.

Notes/Comments:

Demonstrations for [z]

Place: Alveolar

First Method

Objects: None

Instructions:

1. Instruct the student, "Please stick out your tongue."
2. Once the tongue is out, for [s] with the tongue tip raised ask the student to pull the tongue back to feel the bump on the roof of the mouth behind the two front teeth. For [s] with the tongue tip down, ask the student to pull the tongue back to feel the little bump behind the two lower teeth.

Second Method

Objects: Q-tip, peanut butter or other favored food

Instructions:

1. Instruct the student, "Please open your mouth."
2. Once the mouth is open, with Q-tip dab a little peanut butter or other favorite food on alveolar ridge (for tongue tip raised [s]) or behind lower front teeth (for tongue tip lowered [s]).
3. Ask the student to touch the food with the tongue tip.

Manner: Fricative

First Method

Objects: Strip of paper or a feather

Instructions:

1. Place a strip of paper, a feather, or the student's hand held in front of your mouth while you produce several long voiceless fricatives.
2. Draw attention to the "hissing" quality and continuous nature of the sounds.

Second Method

Objects: A small paper flower on end of a pencil

Instructions: Tape a small paper flower on the end of a pencil and encourage the student to move the flower in the wind.

Third Method

Objects: None

Instructions: Run your finger or the student's finger down the student's arm while making several long voiceless fricatives to demonstrate the "hissing" quality and length of fricatives.

Voicing: Voiced

First Method

Objects: None

Instructions: Instruct the student to listen to and identify the difference between a voiceless and voiced [a].

Second Method

Objects: None

Instructions: Place the student's hands over the ears and instruct him or her to hum, which heightens the sensation of vocal cord vibration.

Third Method

Objects: None

Instructions: If the student is able to produce a voiced and voiceless fricative, ask him or her to cover the ears and make these sounds. Alternatively, the student is asked to make [h] and [a].

Fourth Method

Objects: None

Instructions: You and the student place one hand on your throat and the other on the student's throat while making voiced and voiceless sounds together, telling each other when the voicing goes on and off.

Fifth Method

Objects: Pencil, small piece of paper or small paper flower

Instructions: If the student is able to produce a voiced and voiceless oral stop, attach a small piece of paper or a paper flower to the end of a tongue depressor or pencil and ask the student to "make the paper (or flower) move." The paper is more likely to move when a voiceless consonant is produced than when a voiced consonant is produced (be careful in providing instructions to the student, however, because a strongly articulated voiced oral stop will also move the flower).

Phonetic Placement and Shaping Techniques for [z]

To facilitate [z], follow the steps for [s] but also use demonstrations to instruct the student to turn on the voice box.

Shell for Speech Exercises

Student's Name: _____

Date: _____

Treatment Sound: _____

Word List: Student Responses:

1. _____

2. _____

3. _____

4. _____

5. _____

6. _____

7. _____

8. _____

9. _____

10. _____

Total Correct: _____/_____

Comments:

Imitation

Student's Name: _____

Date: _____

Treatment Sound: _____

Goal: Have the student repeat the word after you.

Instructions to Student: "You are going to hear a word with our sound. Please say it after me. Here's an example. I say *sat*, and then you say *sat*."

Word List:	Student Responses:
Zoo	1. _____
Zip	2. _____
Zero	3. _____
Zigzag	4. _____
Zipper	5. _____
Zach	6. _____
Zest	7. _____
Czar	8. _____
Zip code	9. _____
Zoom	10. _____

Total Correct: _____/_____

Comments:

Minimal Pairs

Student's Name: _____

Date: _____

Treatment Sound: _____

Goal: Have the student first say the word with the treatment sound, then say the rhyming word, and then say the word with the treatment sound.

Instructions to Student: "You are going to hear a word that begins with our sound. Please say the word, then replace our sound with another sound to make the word have a different meaning, and then say the word with our sound again. Here's an example. I say *seal*. You say *seal*, then change [s] to [w] to make *wheel*, and then say *seal* again. Like this: *Seal. Wheel. Seal.*"

Word List: Student Responses:

Word List		Student Responses
Zoo	new	1. _____
Zap	tap	2. _____
Zipper	ripper	3. _____
Zen	hen	4. _____
Zeal	meal	5. _____
Zip	hip	6. _____
Zapped	tapped	7. _____
Z	pea	8. _____
Zinc	pink	9. _____
Zest	best	10. _____

Total Correct: _____ / _____

Comments:

Deletion

Student's Name: _____

Date: _____

Treatment Sound: _____

Goal: Have the student first say the word with the treatment sound, then without the treatment sound, and then with the treatment sound.

Instructions to Student: "You are going to hear a word with our sound. Please say the word, and then say it with our sound deleted, and then say it with our sound included. Here's an example. I say *red*. You say *red*, then *Ed*, then *red*. Like this: *Red. Ed. Red.*"

Word List:

		Student Responses:
Zoo	oo	1. _____
Czar	R	2. _____
Z	E	3. _____
Zen	N	4. _____
Zone	own	5. _____
Zinc	ink	6. _____
Zeal	eel	7. _____
Zion	ion	8. _____
		9. _____
		10. _____

Total Correct: _____ / _____

Comments:

Self-Correction

Student's Name: _____

Date: _____

Treatment Sound: _____

Goal: Have the student say the word three times, self-correcting if errors in the treatment sound occur.

Instructions to Student: "You are going to hear a word with our sound. Please say the word three times, listening to how you say our sound and changing it to make it correctly if you say it incorrectly. Here's an example. I say *cheese*, and then you say *cheese* three times, listening to how you say our sound and changing it to make it correctly if you say it incorrectly. Like this: *Cheese. Cheese. Cheese.*"

Word List: **Student Responses:**

Zoo   1. _____

Zip   2. _____

Zero   3. _____

Zigzag   4. _____

Zipper   5. _____

Zach   6. _____

Zest   7. _____

Czar   8. _____

Zip code   9. _____

Zoom   10. _____

Total Correct: _____ / _____

Comments:

Old Way/New Way

Student's Name: _____

Date: _____

Treatment Sound: _____

Goal: Have the student say the word the new way, the old way, and then the new way again.

Instructions to Student: "You are going to hear a word with our sound. Please say the word, then say it the old way you used to say our sound, and then say it the new way you say our sound. Here's an example. I say *thin*. You say *thin*, then **in*, and then *thin*. Like this: *Thin. *in. Thin.*"

Note: Replace * with the way the student used to say the sound.

Word List:	**Student Responses:**
Zoo	1. _____
Zip	2. _____
Zero	3. _____
Zigzag	4. _____
Zipper	5. _____
Zach	6. _____
Zest	7. _____
Czar	8. _____
Zip code	9. _____
Zoom	10. _____

Total Correct: _____ / _____

Comments:

Similar Sound

Student's Name: _____

Date: _____

Treatment Sound: _____

Goal: Have the student first say the word with the treatment sound, then with the most similar sound the student can make, and then with the treatment sound again.

Instructions to Student: "You are going to hear a word with our sound. Please say the word, then replace our sound with _____*, and then say the word with our sound. Here's an example. I say *sun*. You say *sun*, then **un*, and then *sun* again. Like this: *Sun. *un. Sun.*"

Note: Replace * with a sound the student can pronounce that is phonetically similar to the treatment sound.

Word List:	**Student Responses:**
Zoo	1. _____
Zip	2. _____
Zero	3. _____
Zigzag	4. _____
Zipper	5. _____
Zach	6. _____
Zest	7. _____
Czar	8. _____
Zip code	9. _____
Zoom	10. _____

Total Correct: _____ / _____

Comments:

Complete Word List for [z]

Beginning of Words

Single Consonants	Deletions	Minimal Pairs
Zoo	oo	new, shoe, two, moo, goo, boo, chew
Zip		hip, chip, ship, whip, rip, sip, lip
Zero		hero
Zigzag		
Zipper		ripper, nipper
Zach		sack, rack, Mack
Zest		
Czar	R	tar, car, far
Zip code		
Zoom		room, boom, doom
Z	E	pea, me, me, key, D, tea
Zorro		
Zap		tap, zap, rap, map
Zapped		tapped, zapped, rapped, mapped
Zulu		
Zoe		
Zebra		
Zany		
Zen	N	hen, men, Ben, Ken
Zone	own	moan, tone, bone
Zombie		
Zealot		
Zuni		loony, goony
Zephyr		heifer
Zinc	ink	pink, wink, sink, link
Zeal	eel	meal, peel, kneel
Zealot		
Zither		
Zeppelin		
Zing		sing, wing, ping
Zeus		moose, noose
Zurich		
Zion	ion	tie on
Zenith		
Zest		best, west, pest

Consonant Clusters

—

Medial

Single Consonants

Thousand	Freezer	Susan
Daisy	Pisa	Blizzard
Dozen	Tuesday	Zigzag
Rosa	Brazil	Scissors
Muzzle	Pheasant	Busy
Moses	Dessert	Aztec
Rosie	Raisin	Caesar
Wizard	Buzzer	Kansas
Busy	Cheesecake	Prison
Freezing	Daisy	Visor
Boise	Trouser	Puzzle
Muslim	Suzanne	Kansas
Desert	Lizard	Crazy
Nazgul	Music	Thursday
Grizzly	Houses	
Closet	Husband	

Consonant Clusters

Bronze Age	Eavesdrop	Wednesday
Thumbs up	Thumbs down	

All Environments

Thousand	Wizard	Freezer
Daisy	Busy	Pisa
Wednesday	Freezing	Tuesday
Dozen	Boise	Brazil
Rosa	Muslim	Pheasant
Muzzle	Desert	Eavesdrop
Moses	Nazgul	Dessert
Rosie	Grizzly	Raisin
Thumbs up	Closet	Buzzer

All Environments

Cheesecake	Susan	Kansas
Daisy	Bronze Age	Prison
Trouser	Blizzard	Thumbs down
Suzanne	Zigzag	Visor
Lizard	Scissors	Puzzle
Music	Busy	Kansas
Houses	Aztec	Crazy
Husband	Caesar	Thursday

End of Words

Single Consonants

Deletions

Nose	no, know
Buzz	
Rose	row
Cruise	crew
Hose	hoe
Jazz	
Maze	May
Liz	
Samwise	
Snooze	
Graze	gray
Cheese	
Sneeze	
Please	plea
Oz	
News	new
Noise	
Louise	Louie

Consonant Clusters (Plural markers)

Deletion

Tribes	tribe
Bugs	bug
Kings	king
Dimes	dime
Tadpoles	tadpole
Bells	bell

Dwarves	
Seals	seal
Mars	mar
Gloves	glove
Balloons	ballroom
Dreams	dream
Rings	ring
Seashells	seashell
Crabs	crab
Weeds	weed
Balls	ball
Wolves	
Sandals	sandal
Nails	nail
Waves	wave
Ears	ear
Lions	lion
Wings	wing
Drums	drum
Claws	claw
Sea gulls	sea gull
Eggs	egg
Roars	roar
Leopards	leopard
Rinds	rind
Sneakers	sneaker
Ponds	pond
Trolls	troll
Ribbons	ribbon
Whales	whale
Elves	
Crowns	crown
Spareribs	sparerib
Stars	star
Goblins	goblin
Birds	bird
Thumbs	thumb
Tails	tail
Wheels	wheel
Kids	kid
Baggins	
Blackbirds	blackbird
Worlds	world
Dogs	dog

Consonant Clusters (Plural markers)   Deletion

Consonant Clusters (Plural markers)	Deletion
Tears	tear
Hands	hand
Camels	camel
Rugs	rug
Mountains	mountain
Coins	coin
Schoolrooms	schoolroom
Pools	pool
Skateboards	skateboard

Themes for [z]

Themes

Animals   People and Places
Frodo's Journey to Moria   Weekdays
New Oz Stories

Animals   Deletions   Minimal Pairs

Animals	Deletions	Minimal Pairs
Zoo	uh	new, shoe, two, moo, goo, boo, chew
Zebra		
Tadpoles	tadpole	
Muzzle		
Pheasant		
Bugs	bug	
Seals	seal	
Lizard		
Buzz		
Crabs	crab	
Wolves		
Lions	lion	
Wings	wing	
Claws	claw	
Tails	tail	
Eggs	egg	
Roars	roar	
Leopards	leopard	
Sea gulls	sea gull	

Animals	Deletions	Minimal Pairs
Whales	whale	
Birds	bird	
Camels	camel	
Dogs	dog	
Blackbirds	blackbird	

Frodo's Journey to Moria	Deletions	Minimal Pairs
Wizard		
Samwise		
Nazgul		
Baggins		
Rosie		
Dwarves		
Rings	ring	
Blizzard		
Freezing		
Elves		
Pools	pool	
Mountains	mounyain	
Drums	drum	
Crowns	crown	
Kings	king	
Music		
Roars	roar	
Claws	claw	
Maze	May	
Crazy		
Goblins	goblin	

New Oz Stories	Deletions	Minimal Pairs
Kansas		
Oz		
Tribes	tribe	
Zombie		
Worlds	world	
Stars	star	
Dreams	dream	

New Oz Stories	Deletions	Minimal Pairs
Bells	bell	
Prison		
Desert		
Wolves		
Lions	lion	
Wings	wing	
Leopards	leopard	

People and Places	Deletions	Minimal Pairs
Zach		pack, rack, knack
Zorro		
Czar	R	car, tar, mar
Daisy		
Baggins		
Rosa		
Moses		
Louise	Louie	
Aztec		
Suzanne	Sue Ann	
Liz		
Samwise		
Susan		
Caesar		
Rose	row	
Zulu		
Pisa		
Brazil		
Boise		
Kansas		
Oz		
Zeus		moose, noose
Zurich		
Zion	ion	tie on

Weekdays	Deletions	Minimal Pairs
Tuesday		
Wednesday		
Thursday		

Chapter Six

[1]

Definition

[l] is made with the tongue tip raised and touching the mouth roof. Air flows over the sides of the tongue, and the larynx vibrates. The technical definition of [l] is voiced alveolar lateral. Two varieties of [l] exist in English: "light [l]," which occurs at the beginning of syllables, as in **leak** [lik], and "dark [l]," which occurs at the end of syllables, as in **cool** [kul]. In "dark [l]" the back of the tongue is raised in the velar region.

Acquisition

50% of children acquire [l] by 3;6 and 75% of children acquire [l] by 6;0.

Relative Frequency

[l] is ranked 2nd in relative frequency compared to the other late-acquired consonants. It ranks 7th in relative frequency compared to all other English consonants, and its percentage of occurrence compared to all English consonants is 5.6%.

Errors

A common error for [l] is called Gliding—that is, [w] or [j] (glide consonants) substitute for [l] (a liquid consonant). Another common error for [l] is to produce the sound with a wet, slushy quality. Many times a wet, slushy sound occurs when [s] is made with the tongue blade raised instead of the tongue tip.

Key Environments

Light [l]: Before a high front vowel, as in **leaf**
Dark [l]: After a high back vowel at the end of a syllable, as in **call**

Possible Metaphors

Select metaphors based on the aspect of speech that is the focus of therapy.

Tongue placement:	Singing sound (la-la-la)
	Pointy sound (tongue tip pointing to alveolar ridge)
	Bump sound
	Little hill sound
Lateral:	Side sound
Liquid:	Flowing sound
Voicing:	Motor on
	Buzzing sound
	Voice box on sound

Touch Cue

Tip of finger on the middle of the upper lip.

Instruction:

Place the student's finger on the middle of the upper lip.

Initial Screening Test for [l]

Student's Name: _____

Date: _____

Referral: _____

Instructions: Say to the student, "I'm going to say some words. Please say the words after me."
Example: "Dog. Now you say it."

Word	Student*

Beginning

1. Lamp   _____
2. Light   _____
3. Leg   _____
4. Plane   _____
5. Sleep   _____
6. Clip   _____

Medial

7. Sailor   _____
8. Billy   _____
9. Olive   _____

Final

10. Skull   _____
11. Mail   _____
12. Bell   _____
13. Apple   _____
14. Model   _____
15. Muscle   _____

*Suggestion: Transcribe an X if the sound is correct or, if incorrect, phonetically transcribe the error. Ignore errors produced elsewhere in the word.

Comments/Notes:

Stimulability Tests for [l]

Student's Name: _____

Date: _____

Referral: _____

Imitation

   1. lie   _____

   2. low   _____

   3. all   _____

   4. ill   _____

Best Bet Environments

Light [l]:

   1. leaf   _____

   2. leap   _____

Dark [l]: After a high back vowel at the end of a syllable

   1. cool   _____

   2. bull   _____

Favorite Words

Names of family members: _____

Favorite people, heroes, and activities: _____

Phonetic Placement   _____

1. Touch the student's alveolar ridge with a tongue depressor, peanut butter, or lollipop to indicate the place of production for [l].

2. Ask the student to place his or her tongue tip in the place indicated, to relax, and to let air flow out from the sides of the tongue. The resulting sound is voiceless [l].

3. Instruct the student to turn on the voice box, resulting in [l].

Shaping (l) from Interdental (t) ————

1. Ask the student to place the tongue tip between the teeth as for an interdental [t].

2. Lower the student's jaw.

3. Ask the student to slowly draw the tongue tip backward but to keep the tongue tip in contact with the back of the teeth and the ridge behind the two front teeth.

4. Ask the student to say [l], being sure that contact between the tongue and the roof of the mouth is maintained.

Notes/Comments:

Demonstrations for [l]

Place: Alveolar

First Method

Object: None

Instructions:

1. Instruct the student, "Please stick out your tongue."
2. Once the tongue is out, ask the student to pull the tongue back to feel bump on the roof of the mouth behind the two front teeth.

Second Method

Objects: Q-tip, peanut butter or other favored food

Instructions:

1. Instruct the student, "Please open your mouth."
2. One the mouth is open, with Q-tip dab a little peanut butter or other favorite food on alveolar ridge.
3. Ask the student to touch the food with the tongue tip.

Manner: Liquid

First Method

Objects: None

Instructions: Run your or the student's finger down the student's arm while making several long glides or liquids to demonstrate the "flowing" quality and length of this sound.

Second Method

Objects: Strip of paper, a feather, or a small paper flower taped on the end of a pencil

Instructions: Use a strip of paper, a feather, or the hand held in front of the student's mouth while you produce several glides or liquids to draw attention to the "flowing" quality and continuous nature of the sounds. Alternately, tape a small paper flower on the end of a pencil and encourage the student to move the flower in the wind.

Special Demonstration: Lateral Air Flow

First Method

Objects: Drinking straw

Instructions: Place a straw on the groove of the tongue and blow out to demonstrate central emission of air.

Second Method

Objects: Drinking straw

Instructions: Ask the student to breathe in with the tongue as for [s]. Cool air is felt at the central groove. Alternatively, perform the straw technique above, remove the straw, and ask the student to breathe in with the tongue in position for [l]. Cool air should be felt on the sides of the tongue over which the air was emitted. An alternative method is to perform the straw technique above, remove the straws, and ask the student to breathe in.

Voicing: Voiced

First Method

Objects: None

Instructions: Instruct the student to listen to and identify the difference between a voiceless and voiced [a].

Second Method

Objects: None

Instructions: Place the student's hands over the ears and instruct him or her to hum, which heightens the sensation of vocal cord vibration.

Third Method

Objects: None

Instructions: If the student is able to produce a voiced and voiceless fricative, ask him or her to cover the ears and make these sounds. Alternatively, the student is asked to make [h] and [a].

Fourth Method

Objects: None

Instructions: You and the student place one hand on your throat and the other on the student's throat while making voiced and voiceless sounds together, telling each other when the voicing goes on and off.

Fifth Method

Objects: Pencil, small piece of paper or small paper flower

Instructions: If the student is able to produce a voiced and voiceless oral stop, attach a small piece of paper or a paper flower to the end of a tongue depressor or pencil and ask the student to "make the paper (or flower) move." The paper is more likely to move when a voiceless consonant is produced than when a voiced consonant is produced (be careful in providing instructions to the student, however, because a strongly articulated voiced oral stop will also move the flower).

Phonetic Placement and Shaping Techniques for [l]

Phonetic Placement Techniques

Most often, the challenge with [l] is to help the student direct the airflow over the sides of the tongue. These four methods each focus on helping the student achieve lateral airflow. The first three methods focus on [l] in isolation and the fourth focuses on [l] in consonant clusters.

First Method

Objects: Tongue depressor

Instructions:

1. Place a tongue depressor under the student's tongue tip and then raise the tongue tip behind the upper front teeth.
2. Ask the student to say [l] while maintaining contact between the tongue tip and the roof of the mouth. The resulting sound is [l].

Second Method

Objects: Tongue depressor, small dab of peanut butter, or lollipop

Instructions:

1. Touch the student's alveolar ridge with a tongue depressor, peanut butter, or lollipop to indicate the place of production for [l].
2. Ask the student to place the tongue tip in the place indicated, to relax, and to let air flow out from the sides of the tongue. The resulting sound is voiceless [l].
3. Instruct the student to turn on the voice box, resulting in [l].

Third Method

This method works, though the number of steps limits its effectiveness, unless the student has good motivation and attention.

Objects: Small piece of paper, two drinking straws

Instructions:

1. Place a straw midline on the student's tongue groove to demonstrate central air emission. Ask the student to blow out onto an open hand or piece of paper. An alternative (or additional) demonstration of central air emission is to ask the student to prepare the mouth to say [s] but to breathe in. Cool air is felt midline on the upper tongue surface.
2. Next, place a straw in each corner of the student's mouth. Ask the student to breathe out into his or her open hand or on a piece of paper. If an additional demonstration is needed, remove the straws and ask the student to breathe in and to feel the cool air on the sides of the tongue over which the air is emitted. To demonstrate the feel of the air more vividly, ask the student to suck on a piece of peppermint candy for a few minutes before performing the demonstration.
3. After lateral emission of air is obtained, ask the student to place the tongue tip in contact with the roof of the mouth behind the upper front teeth and to blow out over the sides of the tongue. If needed, place straws in the side of the student's mouth while the tongue tip is held in contact with the roof of the mouth.
4. Ask the student to blow air out the side straws, which results in the voiceless [l].
5. Voicing is obtained by asking the student to turn on the voice box. The resulting sound is [l].

Fourth Method

This method is for a student who needs to learn to pronounce [l] in consonant clusters. The method works for consonant clusters in which the other consonant in the cluster is not alveolar—for example, a velar or labial stop.

Objects: None

Instructions:

1. Instruct the student to place the tongue in the position for /l/.
2. Instruct the student to say "blue," resulting in a [bl] consonant cluster.

Shaping Techniques

(l) from (θ) or (ð) ────────────────────────

If a student's speech contains a well-established interdental, this can be converted into [l]. Instead of an interdental, [s] or [z] can be used, though the task is more difficult for most students, because [s] and [z] are harder to see move than the interdental fricatives.

Objects: None

Instructions:

1. Ask the student to place the tongue tip between the teeth as for [ð].
2. Lower the student's jaw.
3. Ask the student to slowly draw the tongue tip backward but to keep the tongue tip in contact with the back of the teeth and the ridge behind the two front teeth.
4. Next, instruct the student to say [l], being sure that contact between the tongue and the roof of the mouth is maintained. If [θ] is used, instruct the student to turn on the voice box.

(l) from (i) or (u) ────────────────────────

This method sounds tricky. It works, though, with selected students.

Objects: None

Instructions:

1. Ask the student to open the mouth as wide as for [a] but to raise the tongue tip as for [i].
2. Ask the student to keep the tongue up as for [i] but to say [a], resulting in a light (alveolar) [l]. (*Note:* For a dark (velar) [l], follow the same steps but ask the student to say [u] instead of [i]).

Shell for Speech Exercises

Student's Name: _____

Date: _____

Treatment Sound: _____

Word List: Student Responses:

                                   1. _____

                                   2. _____

                                   3. _____

                                   4. _____

                                   5. _____

                                   6. _____

                                   7. _____

                                   8. _____

                                   9. _____

                                 10. _____

Total Correct: _____/_____

Comments:

Imitation

Student's Name: _____

Date: _____

Treatment Sound: _____

Goal: Have the student repeat the word after you.

Instructions to Student: "You are going to hear a word with our sound. Please say it after me. Here's an example. I say *sat*, and then you say *sat*."

Word List:	Student Responses:
Log	1. _____
Leather	2. _____
Lick	3. _____
Lock	4. _____
Lake	5. _____
Litter	6. _____
Lump	7. _____
Look	8. _____
Low	9. _____
Lip	10. _____

Total Correct: _____/_____

Comments:

Minimal Pairs

Student's Name: _____

Date: _____

Treatment Sound: _____

Goal: Have the student first say the word with the treatment sound, then say the rhyming word, and then say the word with the treatment sound.

Instructions to Student: "You are going to hear a word that begins with our sound. Please say the word, then replace our sound with another sound to make the word have a different meaning, and then say the word with our sound again. Here's an example. I say *seal*. You say *seal*, then change [s] to [w] to make *wheel*, and then say *seal* again. Like this: *Seal. Wheel. Seal.*"

Word List:		Student Responses:
Low	bow	1. _____
Larry	berry	2. _____
Lair	fair	3. _____
Lock	sock	4. _____
Lamp	ramp	5. _____
Look	book	6. _____
Log	dog	7. _____
Lump	dump	8. _____
Leg	beg	9. _____
Ladder	sadder	10. _____

Total Correct: _____ / _____

Comments:

Deletion

Goal: Have the student first say the word with the treatment sound, then without the treatment sound, and then with the treatment sound.

Instructions to Student: "You are going to hear a word with our sound. Please say the word, and then say it with our sound deleted, and then say it with our sound included. Here's an example. I say *red*. You say *red*, then *Ed*, then *red*. Like this: *Red. Ed. Red.*"

Word List:

Lick	ick	
Lake	ache	
Low	O, oh	
Lion	ion	
Lair	air	
Lamp	amp	
Leg	egg	
Ladder	adder	
Larry	airy	
Lou	uh	

Student Responses:

1. _____
2. _____
3. _____
4. _____
5. _____
6. _____
7. _____
8. _____
9. _____
10. _____

Total Correct: _____ / _____

Comments:

Self-Correction

Student's Name: _____

Date: _____

Treatment Sound: _____

Goal: Have the student say the word three times, self-correcting if errors in the treatment sound occur.

Instructions to Student: "You are going to hear a word with our sound. Please say the word three times, listening to how you say our sound and changing it to make it correctly if you say it incorrectly. Here's an example. I say *cheese*, and then you say *cheese* three times, listening to how you say our sound and changing it to make it correctly if you say it incorrectly. Like this: *Cheese. Cheese. Cheese.*"

Word List:	Student Responses:
Log	1. _____
Leather	2. _____
Lick	3. _____
Lock	4. _____
Lake	5. _____
Litter	6. _____
Lump	7. _____
Look	8. _____
Low	9. _____
Lip	10. _____

Total Correct: _____ / _____

Comments:

Old Way/New Way

Student's Name: _____

Date: _____

Treatment Sound: _____

Goal: Have the student say the word the new way, the old way, and then the new way again.

Instructions to Student: "You are going to hear a word with our sound. Please say the word, then say it the old way you used to say our sound, and then say it the new way you say our sound. Here's an example. I say *thin*. You say *thin*, then **in*, and then *thin*. Like this: *Thin. *in. Thin.*"

Note: Replace * with the way the student used to say the sound.

Word List:	Student Responses:
Log	1. _____
Leather	2. _____
Lick	3. _____
Lock	4. _____
Lake	5. _____
Litter	6. _____
Lump	7. _____
Look	8. _____
Low	9. _____
Lip	10. _____

Total Correct: _____ / _____

Comments:

Similar Sound

Student's Name: _____

Date: _____

Treatment Sound: _____

Goal: Have the student first say the word with the treatment sound, then with the most similar sound the student can make, and then with the treatment sound again.

Instructions to Student: "You are going to hear a word with our sound. Please say the word, then replace our sound with _____*, and then say the word with our sound. Here's an example. I say *sun*. You say *sun*, then **un*, and then *sun* again. Like this: *Sun. *un. Sun.*"

Note: Replace * with a sound the student can pronounce that is phonetically similar to the treatment sound.

Word List:	Student Responses:
Log	1. _____
Leather	2. _____
Lick	3. _____
Lock	4. _____
Lake	5. _____
Litter	6. _____
Lump	7. _____
Look	8. _____
Low	9. _____
Lip	10. _____

Total Correct: _____ / _____

Comments:

Complete Word List for [l]

Beginning of Words

Single Consonants	Deletions	Minimal Pairs
Log		dog, hog, bog
Leather		feather, heather, weather
Lick	ick	sick, tick, wick, pick, kick, thick
Lock		sock, knock, rock
Lake	ache	bake, cake
Litter		sitter
Lump		dump, pump
Look		book, cook, hook
Low	O, oh	bow, sew, foe, no, know
Lip		zip, rip, dip, whip, sip, chip, ship, hip
Lettuce		bet us
Lagoon		
Lion	ion	
Legolas		
Lair	air	fair, hair, mare, tear, chair
Lamp	amp	ramp, camp, damp
Light		night, write, white, bite, fight, kite
Leg	egg	beg, Meg,
Ladder	adder	sadder, madder
Line		sign, mine, line, pine, nine
List		mist, wrist, kissed, hissed
Letter		better, setter
Lantern		
Larry	airy	berry, Barry, merry, cherry
Lou	oo	new, chew, Sue, Rue, two
Leech	each	beech, reach
Ladies		
Lemon		
Lei	A	day, bay, say, gray, hay
Lime	I'm	dime, rhyme, mime
Lie	I, eye	buy, guy, sigh, rye, die, fly, sigh, pie
Leopard		
Lawrence		
Long		song, wrong

Single Consonants	Deletions	Minimal Pairs
Late	ate	date, rate, gate, hate, bait
Leonard		
Lava		Java
Lawn	awn	Shawn
Leak	eek	beak, meek, peak
Llama		
Lois		
Lobster		
Luke		nuke, kook
Leap		peep, reap, seep
Laugh		calf, half
Leash		
Lisp		wisp
Limp	imp	wimp, gimp
Lynn	in	win, sin, tin
Lincoln		
Love		dove, shove
Lumber		number
Life		knife
Leaf		chief, thief
Lung		sung, rung, hung
Lamb	am	Sam, ram, ham
Lace	ace	race, chase, face
Loaf	oaf	
Land	and	sand, band
Limb		gym Jim, him, rim
Lance		dance, chance
Lucy		juicy
Luggage		
Lad	add	bad, mad, sad
Load	ode	code, node, bode
Lazy		daisy
Lunch		bunch, munch, hunch
Link	ink	sink, rink, mink
Lid	id	hid, bid, mid
Least	east	beast
Like	Ike	Mike, bike, pike
London		
Lane		mane, sane, bane
Lone	own	tone, moan
Label	able	sable, Mabel
Lap		nap, cap

Single Consonants	Deletions	Minimal Pairs
Locker		succor
Lame	aim	game, same, name
Lace	ace	race, case, base
Lady		Sadie
Lye	I, eye	tie, die, sigh

Consonant Clusters	Deletions	Minimal Pairs

(pl)

Plane	pain, pane	
Plywood		
Plants	pants	
Plant food		
Play	pay	pray
Pluto		
Planet		
Plank		prank
Plato		
Platoon		
Plowed		proud
Please	peas	
Plastic		
Plaza		
Plymouth		
Pliers		
Plate	pate	
Playground		
Plum		
Placard		

(kl)

Clark		quark
Clip	Kip	quip
Club	cub	
Classroom		
Class	Cass	crass
Clock	cock	crock
Clipper		
Clap	cap	crap

Consonant Clusters	Deletions	Minimal Pairs
Clifford		
Clay	K	Kray
Clamshell		
Clerk	Kirk	quirk
Cliff		
Clever		
Cluck		
Cloud	cowed	crowd
Clippers	kippers	
Clam	cam	cram
Clover		
Clown		crown
Claw	caw	craw
Climb		crime

(bl)

Black	back	
Blue	boo	brew
Blind	bind	
Blizzard		
Blossom		
Bleed	bead	breed
Blackbird		
Block		Brock
Blindfold		
Blender	bender	
Blank	bank	
Bloodhound		
Blackmail		
Blood	bud	

(gl)

Glove		grove
Glass	gas	grass
Glacier		
Glenn		
Glad		grad
Glitter		
Globe		
Glider		

Consonant Clusters	Deletions	Minimal Pairs
Glow	go	grow
Glue	goo	grew
Gloomy		
Glasses	gasses	grasses

(fl)

Floor	four	
Flashbulb		
Flag		
Fly	fie	fry
Flood	food	
Flight	fight	fright
Flagstaff		
Flat	fat	frat
Flipper		
Flash		
Flea	fee	free
Flour		
Florist	forest	
Flab	fab	
Flame		frame
Flip		
Flower		

(sl)

Slip	sip	skip
Slaw	saw	
Sledding		
Slide	side	spied
Slap	sap	
Sleigh bells		
Sleet	seat	skeet, sweet
Slug		
Sleep	seep	steep, sweep
Slop	sop	stop, swap
Sleeve	sieve	Steve
Slicing		spicing
Slipper	sipper	skipper
Sled dog		
Slum	sum	scum

Consonant Clusters	Deletions	Minimal Pairs
Sliver		
Sled	said	sped
Sloth		
Sleigh	say	stay, spay, sway
Sling	sing	sting, swing
Sleepy		
Slurp		

(spl)

Splash		
Splinter		sprinter
Splendid		
Splay	play	
Splashdown		
Splatter		
Splurge		
Splice		
Spleen		
Splat		
Split		
Splutter		
Splint		sprint
Splotchy		
Splashy		
Splendor		

All Consonant Clusters	Deletions	Minimal Pairs
Plane	pain, pane	
Glasses	gasses	grasses
Plants	pants	
Sleep	seep	sweep, steep
Pluto		
Slicing		spicing
Plank		prank
Platoon		
Clip	Kip	quip
Plywood		
Plowed		proud

All Consonant Clusters	Deletions	Minimal Pairs
Clark		quark
Play	pay	pray, prey
Clipper	Kipper	
Slop	sop	stop, swap
Club	cub	
Classroom		
Plastic		
Class	Cass	crass
Clock	cock	crock
Plant food		
Clap	cap	crap
Glue	goo	grew
Globe		
Clifford		
Clay	K	Kray
Slipper	sipper	skipper
Clamshell		
Slap	sap	
Flab	fab	
Sleigh bells		
Planet		
Sled dog		
Slum	sum	scum
Clever		
Blossom		
Cluck		
Cloud	cowed	crowd
Sleeve	sieve	Steve
Clippers	kippers	
Clam	cam	cram
Sleet	seat	skeet, sweet
Clover		
Gloomy		
Slug		
Clown		crown
Plato		
Claw	caw	
Playground		
Climb		crime
Black	back	
Sled	said	sped

All Consonant Clusters	Deletions	Minimal Pairs
Blue	boo	brew
Plymouth		
Blind	bind	
Clerk	Kirk	
Flip		
Pliers		
Flower		
Blizzard		
Plate	pate	
Bleed	bead	breed
Glass	gas	grass
Block		Brock
Flood	food	
Florist	forest	
Slide	side	spied
Cliff		
Sliver		
Blood	bud	
Fly	fie	fry
Plaza		
Glove		
Bloodhound		
Glacier		
Flight	fight	fright
Glenn		
Splashdown		
Glitter		
Blank	bank	
Globe		
Blackbird		
Glider		
Blender	bender	
Glow	go	grow
Splash		
Floor	four	
Splinter		
Flashbulb		
Glad		
Flag		
Splendid		
Sleigh	say	stray, stay, sway

All Consonant Clusters	Deletions	Minimal Pairs
Sleepy		
Blindfold		
Flagstaff		
Sling	sing	sting, swing
Flat	fat	frat
Flipper		
Blackmail		
Flash		
Slurp		
Flea	fee	free
Flour		
Plum		
Flame	fame	frame
Slip	sip	skip
Slaw	saw	
Sledding		
Please	peas	
Sloth		
Placard		

Medial

Single Consonants

Sailor	Ireland	Dallas
Billy	Chile	Sailor
Olive	Kelly	Pillow
Smiling	Cellar	Aileen
Ceylon	Julie	Eyelash
Ballet	Toilet	Bowling
Valley	Jailer	Albert
Eyelid	Zulu	Boulder
Galleon	Cello	Melbourne
Boiling	Shelley	Gallon
Chilly	Collar	Jello
Gimli	Children	Chilly
Collar	Alley	Police
Ruler	Island	Ceiling
Palace	Balloon	Hilly
Delhi	Salad	

Consonant Clusters

Airplane	Milkshake	Burglar
Apply	School bus	Cornflake
Applaud	Wobbling	Snowflake
Cobbler	Giggling	Goblin
Douglas	England	Stiffly
Duckling	Wildfire	Wrestler
Ticklish	Gobbler	Asleep
Weekly	Cornflakes	Nicely
Bubbling	Ugly	
Album	Toddler	

All Environments

Cobbler	Chile	Wrestler
Sailor	Weekly	Island
Bubbling	Kelly	Cornflake
Billy	Cellar	Balloon
Olive	Gobbler	Apply
Smiling	Julie	Salad
Album	Toilet	Dallas
Applaud	Jailer	Burglar
Ceylon	Duckling	Sailor
Ballet	Zulu	Pillow
Valley	Cello	Aileen
Eyelid	Ticklish	Stiffly
Galleon	Shelley	Eyelash
Boiling	Collar	Bowling
Chilly	Children	Albert
Airplane	Alley	Boulder
Gimli	Wobbling	Nicely
Douglas	Giggling	Melbourne
Collar	England	Gallon
Ruler	Wildfire	Jello
Milkshake	Cornflakes	Asleep
Palace	Ugly	Chilly
School bus	Toddler	Police
Delhi	Snowflake	Ceiling
Ireland	Goblin	Hilly

End of Words

Single Consonants	*Deletions*
Roll	row
Wheel	whee
Rail	ray
Tile	tie
Skull	
Mail	may
Towel	
Bell	
Dial	die
Seal	sea, see
Boil	boy
Mall	
Snail	
Seashell	
Hole	ho
Veil	
Pile	pie
Mole	
Peel	pea
Spool	
Cell	
School	
Cool	
Bowl	bow
Nail	
Drill	
Troll	toll
Pail	pay
Mel	
Bill	
Goal	go
Eel	E
Gail	gay
Bull	
Baseball	
Coal	
Pill	
Ball	
Churchill	

Single Consonants	Deletions
Steal	
Fall	
April	
Drool	
Doll	
Daniel	
Jail	J
Phil	
Carol	
Yell	
Steel	
Cheryl	
Hall	
Beach ball	
Seagull	
Brazil	
Wall	
Tadpole	
Hotel	
Oatmeal	
Jackal	
Whale	way
Cartwheel	
North Pole	

Consonant Clusters   Deletions

(pl)

Apple
People
Scalpel
Steeple
Maple
People

(bl)

Cable
Bible
Fable

Consonant Clusters   *Deletions*

Hubble
Bubble
Scrabble
Pebble

(dl)

Model
Pedal
Candle
Cradle

(gl)

Eagle
Beagle
Bugle

(fl)

Cheerful
Eiffel
Sniffle

Velar Nasal (l)

Jungle
Bungle

(nl)

Funnel
Colonel
Tunnel
Kernel

(kl)

Jackal
Ankle
Buckle
Knuckle
Snorkel

Consonant Clusters   Deletions

(dl)

Devil

(sl)

Missile
Castle
Fossil
Pencil
Muscle
Capsule

(ʃ) + (l)

Marshal

(lv)

Twelve

(lt)

Salt	sought
Belt	bet
Vault	
Bolt	
Bank vault	

(ld)

Child	chide
Donald	
World	word
Old	ode
Gold	goad
Stronghold	
Bald	
Field	feed
Windshield	
Arnold	

Consonant Clusters	Deletions

(lf)

Elf	F
Werewolf	
Golf	
Wolf	woof
Shelf	chef
Rudolph	
Gandolf	

(lb)

Light bulb
DeKalb

(lm)

Elm	M
Helm	hem

(lp)

Kelp
Alp
Scalp

(lk)

Milk
Silk
Elk
Hulk

Consonant + Syllabic (l)

Apple
Model
Muscle
People
Beagle
Steeple
Bugle

Consonant Clusters	**Deletions**
Maple	
People	
Fossil	
Cable	
Scalpel	
Bible	
Pencil	
Hubble	
Snorkel	
Bubble	
Ankle	
Pedal	
Candle	
Knuckle	
Cradle	
Eagle	
Cheerful	
Buckle	
Eiffel	
Sniffle	
Jungle	
Fable	
Bungle	
Funnel	
Pebble	
Colonel	
Missile	
Tunnel	
Kernel	
Jackal	
Scrabble	
Devil	
Castle	
Capsule	
Marshal	

(l) + Consonant

Stronghold	
Twelve	
Salt	sought
Hulk	

Consonant Clusters	*Deletions*
Vault	
Light bulb	
Bolt	
Bank vault	
Child	chide
Shelf	chef
Donald	
Bald	
World	word
Belt	bet
Gold	goad
Windshield	
Arnold	
Gandolf	
Elk	
Alp	
Elf	F
Werewolf	
Silk	
Wolf	woof
Rudolph	
Old	ode
DeKalb	
Golf	
Elm	M
Field	feed
Scalp	
Helm	hem
Kelp	
Milk	

Themes for (l)

Themes:

Northern Places	Make a Healthy Lunch
Day at the Beach	People to See
Sea Voyage to Old Hawaii	Places to Go
Let's Cook	Animals
Lord of the Rings	Make Up a Fairy Tale

Northern Places	Deletions	Minimal Pairs
Chilly		
Elk		
Rudolph		
Sled	said	sped
Sled dog		
Sleigh bells		
Sleet	seat	skeet, sweet
Glacier		
Blizzard		
North Pole		
Cool	coo	
Wolf	woof	
Wolves		
Sledding		
Sleigh	say	stay, spay, spray
Snowflake		

Day at the Beach	Deletions	Minimal Pairs
Lobster		
Salt		bought, taught
Snorkel		
Pebble		
Splash		
Flipper		
Clamshell		
Beach ball		
Seagull		
Pail	pay	
Towel		
Seal	sea, see	sea, see
Snail		
Seashell		
Kelp		
Whale	way	
Eel	E	

Sea Voyage to Old Hawaii	**Deletions**	**Minimal Pairs**
Sailor		
Galleon		
Clipper	Kipper	
Lei	A	say, pay, may
Boil	boy	
Lava		Java
Hilly		
Island		
Boiling		

Let's Cook	**Deletions**	**Minimal Pairs**
Lettuce		
Lemon		
Lime	I'm	dime, rhyme, mime
Milk		
Apple		
Bubbling		
Cobbler		
Boil	boy	
Slicing		spicing
Slaw	saw	
Flour		
Glass	gas	grass
Blender	bender	
Clam	cam	cram
Plate	pate	
Plum		
Lunch		bunch, munch, hunch
Lid	id	hid, bid, mid
Like	Ike	Mike, bike, pike
Peel	pea	
Loaf	oaf	
Olive		
Bowl	bow	
Chile		
Salad		
Jello		
Roll	row	
Oatmeal		

Let's Cook	Deletions	Minimal Pairs
Duckling		
Cornflakes		

Lord of the Rings	Deletions	Minimal Pairs
Gandolf		
Elrond		
Gimli		
Legolas		
Gollum		
Elf	F	
Wolf	woof	
Wolves		
Eagle		beagle
Troll		stroll
Trolls		
Goblins		
Lady		Sadie
Lad	add	bad, mad, sad

Make a Healthy Lunch	Deletions	Minimal Pairs
Lettuce		
Lemon		
Milk		
Apple		
Slicing	spicing	
Glass	gas	grass
Plate	pate	
Plum		slum
Peel	pea	
Loaf	oaf	
Olive		
Bowl	bow	
Salad		
Roll	row	

People to See	Deletions	Minimal Pairs
Kelly		
Gimli		
Lance		dance, chance
Lucy		juicy
Gandolf		
Lynn	in	win, sin, tin
Billy		
Lincoln		
Leonard		
Larry	airy	berry, Barry, merry, cherry
Lou	oo	two, new, boo, goo, new, chew, Sue, Rue, two
Gail	gay	
Julie		
Legolas		
Lawrence		
Gollum		
Lois		
Luke		nuke, kook
Elrond		
Zulu		
Shelley		
Aileen		
Arnold		
Donald		
Albert		
Glenn		
Cliff		
Clifford		
Clark		quark
Plato		
Douglas		
(The) Hulk		
Kelly		
(The) Devil		
Billy		
Mel		
Bill		
Churchill		
April		
Daniel		
Phil		
Carol		
Cheryl		

Places to Go	Deletions	Minimal Pairs
Ceylon		
Ireland		
Dallas		
England		
Delhi		
London		
Ireland		
Chile		
Dallas		
Brazil		
Pluto		
(The) Hubble		
Plymouth		
Flagstaff		
Boulder		
Melbourne		
Eiffel (Tower)		
DeKalb		

Animals	Deletions	Minimal Pairs
Leech	each	beach, reach
Lair	air	fair, hair, mare, tear, chair
Lion	ion	
Leopard		
Lick	ick	sick, tick, wick, pick, kick, thick
Llama		
Lamb		Sam, ram, ham
Eel	E	
Eagle		
Beagle		
Gobbler		
Sloth		
Flea	fee	free
Claw	caw	
Tadpole		
Jackal		
Blackbird		
Slug		
Wolf	woof	
Wolves		

Make Up a Fairy Tale	**Deletions**	**Minimal Pairs**
Valley		
Lake	ache	bake, cake
Lock		sock, knock, rock
Lamp	amp	ramp, camp, damp
Light		night, write, white, bite, fight, kite
Lawn		Shawn
Elf	F	
Castle		
Tunnel		
Werewolf		
Steeple		
Ugly		
Goblin		
Lame	aim	game, same, name
Lace	ace	race, case, base
Lazy		daisy
Lye	I, eye	tie, die, sigh
England		
Flower		
Flame	fame	frame
Jail	J	
Cell		
Lady		Sadie
Lad	add	bad, mad, sad
Veil		
Slipper	sipper	
Fable		
Lagoon		

Chapter Seven

Vocalic

[r]

Definition

Vocalic [r] is a vowel rather than a consonant, and is included in this book because often the road to a good [r] leads through first learning to make vocalic [r]. Vocalic [r] is heard in the words *heard*, *butter*, and *girl*. As with its consonant counterpart (called consonantal [r] or simply [r]), it is produced in either of two ways. In the first way, called bunched, the lips are rounded slightly, the tongue tip lowered, and the tongue body bunched up near the area of the palate. In the second way, called retroflex, the lips are rounded slightly and tongue tip is raised and raised either toward the alveolar ridge or curled back toward the alveolar ridge. In both varieties of vocalic [r], the sides of the tongue touch the insides of the teeth about halfway back. Both bunched and retroflex types of vocalic [r] can result in a good sound, though the author's clinical experience is that more students find the bunched variation somewhat easier to learn than the retroflex one. For both types of vocalic [r], the vocal folds are vibrating and the tongue root is retracted, creating a contraction in the pharynx. The technical definition of vocalic [r] is a mid-central rounded rhoticized vowel.

Acquisition

Vocalic [r] is acquired by 50% of children by 3;6 and 75% of children by 5;6.

Relative Frequency

—

Errors

The most common error is deleting the [r] part of the vowel, resulting in words such as *fur*, *fare*, and *fear* being pronounced *fu*, *fa*, *fe*, respectively.

Key Environments

In a word consisting of a single stressed syllable, as in *girl*.

Possible Metaphors

The best metaphor usually focuses on the way vocalic [r] closes (ends) the vowel.

[r] quality:	Mad dog or growling-tiger sound (grr)
	Arm-wrestling sound (errr)
	Pirate sound (aar)
Tongue placement:	Tongue-tip flat sound (bunched)
	Tongue-tip up sound (retroflex)
Voicing:	Motor on
	Buzzing sound
	Voice box on sound

Touch Cue

Palm down and finger tips curled down (bunched) or palm up and finger tips curled up (retroflex).

Instructions:

Place the student's hand beside the mouth.

Initial Screening Test for Vocalic [r]

Student's Name: _____

Date: _____

Referral: _____

Instructions: Say to the student, "I'm going to say some words. Please say the words after me."
Example: "Dog. Now you say it."

Word	Student*

Open

1. Grocer   _____
2. Racer   _____
3. Sister   _____
4. Monster   _____
5. Chester   _____

Closed

6. Bird   _____
7. Shirt   _____
8. Burn   _____
9. Hurl   _____
10. Nurse   _____

*Suggestion: Transcribe an X if the sound is correct or, if incorrect, phonetically transcribe the error. Ignore errors produced elsewhere in the word.

Comments/Notes:

Stimulability Tests for Vocalic (r)

Student's Name: _____

Date: _____

Referral: _____

Imitation

  1. h<u>er</u>   _____

  2. c<u>ur</u>l   _____

Best Bet Environments

In a word consisting of a single stressed syllable

  1. h<u>er</u>   _____

  2. g<u>ir</u>l   _____

Favorite Words

Names of family members: _____

Favorite people, heroes, and activities: _____

Phonetic Placement   _____

Instruct the student to growl like a tiger (grrr). Alternatively, ask the student to make the "arm wrestling sound" ([rrr]) while arm wrestling with the clinician.

Vocalic (r) (retroflex) from (ð)

1. Ask the student to place the tongue as for [ð].

2. Ask the student to quickly draw the tongue tip back and slightly up, resulting in vocalic [r].

Notes/Comments:

Demonstrations for Vocalic [r]

Place: Alveolar

First Method

Objects: None

Instructions:

1. Instruct the student, "Please stick out your tongue."
2. Once the tongue is out, for vocalic [r] with the tongue tip lowered, ask the student to pull the tongue back and touch the gums below the two lower front teeth. For vocalic [r] with the tongue tip raised, ask the student to pull back the tongue to feel the bump on the roof of the mouth behind the two upper front teeth.

Second Method

Objects: Q-tip, peanut butter or other favored food

Instructions:

1. Instruct the student, "Please open your mouth."
2. One the mouth is open, with Q-tip dab a little peanut butter or other favorite food on alveolar ridge (for tongue tip raised vocalic [r]) or behind lower front teeth (for tongue tip lowered vocalic [r]).
3. Ask the student to touch the food with the tongue tip.

Manner: Liquid

First Method

Objects: None

Instructions: Run your or the student's finger down the student's arm while making several long glides or liquids to demonstrate the "flowing" quality and length of this sound.

Second Method

Objects: Strip of paper, a feather, or a small paper flower taped on the end of a pencil

Instructions: Use a strip of paper, a feather, or the hand held in front of the student's mouth while you produce several glides or liquids to draw attention to the "flowing" quality and continuous nature of the sounds. Alternately, tape a small paper flower on the end of a pencil and encourage the student to move the flower in the wind.

Special Demonstration: Bunched

A Q-tip, small piece of candy, or other favored food sometimes is helpful in demonstrating where to place the tongue tip.

First Method

Objects: None

Instructions: Ask the student to place the tongue tip behind the lower front teeth and to raise the body of the tongue toward the mouth roof.

Second Method

Objects: Q-tip or small piece of candy or other favored food

Instructions:

1. Touch behind the student's lower front teeth with a Q-tip to demonstrate where the tongue tip should be placed. Alternatively, place a small piece of candy or other favored food behind the lower front teeth and ask the student to hold it there with the tongue tip.
2. Once this is achieved, ask the student to raise the tongue body toward the mouth roof.

Special Demonstration: Retroflex

A Q-tip, small piece of candy, or other favored food sometimes is helpful in demonstrating where to place the tongue tip.

Method

Objects: None

Instructions:

1. Ask the student to place the tongue tip behind the upper front teeth.
2. Ask the student to curl the tongue backward without touching the roof of the mouth until it cannot go back farther.

Sides of Tongue (Bunched and Retroflex): Vocalic and Consonantal [r]

A good [r] often is more easily achieved if the student is encouraged to say the sound while keeping the sides of the tongue touching the insides of the teeth. The following simple demonstration can be practiced in isolation or as part of the bunched and retroflex demonstrations.

First Method

Objects: None

Instructions:

1. Tell the student that his or her tongue is sleepy and wants to rest.
2. Instruct the student to let the tongue spread out in "its bed" until it is touching the insides of the teeth.

Second Method

Objects: Q-tip, candy, or other favored food

Instructions:

1. Touch the inside teeth with a Q-tip or some favored food to demonstrate where the tongue should go.
2. Tell the student that his or her tongue is sleepy and wants to rest.
3. Instruct the student to let the tongue spread out in "its bed" until it is touching the insides of the teeth.

Voicing: Voiced

First Method

Objects: None

Instructions: Instruct the student to listen to and identify the difference between a voiceless and voiced [a].

Second Method

Objects: None

Instructions: Place the student's hands over the ears and instruct him or her to hum, which heightens the sensation of vocal cord vibration.

Third Method

Objects: None

Instructions: If the student is able to produce a voiced and voiceless fricative, ask him or her to cover the ears and make these sounds. Alternatively, the student is asked to make [h] and [a].

Fourth Method

Objects: None

Instructions: You and the student place one hand on your throat and the other on the student's throat while making voiced and voiceless sounds together, telling each other when the voicing goes on and off.

Fifth Method

Objects: Pencil, small piece of paper or small paper flower

Instructions: If the student is able to produce a voiced and voiceless oral stop, attach a small piece of paper or a paper flower to the end of a tongue depressor or pencil and ask the student to "make the paper (or flower) move." The paper is more likely to move when a voiceless consonant is produced than when a voiced consonant is produced (be careful in providing instructions to the student, however, because a strongly articulated voiced oral stop will also move the flower).

Phonetic Placement and Shaping Techniques for Vocalic [r]

Phonetic Placement Techniques

The first three techniques are simple and quick. If they don't work, try the fourth or fifth methods.

First Method (retroflex or bunched)

Objects: None

Instructions: Ask the student to growl like a tiger (grrr). Alternatively, ask the student to make the "arm-wrestling sound" (rrr) while you and the student arm wrestle.

Second Method (retroflex)

I like this method—it is simple, quick, needs no objects, and is good both for vocalic [r] and for shaping vocalic [r] into consonant [r]. It comes from Gillian Fleming of Dunedin, New Zealand, who posted it on Caroline Bowen's Web site and kindly consented for it to be presented in this book.

Objects: None

Instructions:

1. Instruct the student that for this sound it is the tongue that does the work, and that the lips need to be "out of the road" in a half-smile so that the upper and lower teeth can be seen.
2. Model a long vocalic [r], and then ask the student to curl the tongue back to copy your model. Allow the student to move the tongue around until a perfect production is reached. If the student has difficulty, liken the sound to "a car starting on a frosty morning" to elicit a growly *rrrrr* sound.
3. Once vocalic [r] is produced, ask the student to "feel" where the tongue is.
4. Once established in isolation, practice vocalic [r] in syllables, such as *rrah* and *rrrye*.
5. Once *rrah* and *rrye* have been achieved, instruct the student to place the tongue tip up and back until the correct [r] is achieved and then have the student say *ring*.

Third Method (retroflex or bunched) _____

This method works by stretching and spreading the sides of the mouth. Somewhat surprisingly, for some students it places the tongue in just the right position to make vocalic [r].

Objects: Thin drinking straw

Instructions:

1. Ask the student to "make a face" by hooking the first finger of each hand in the corner of the mouth and stretching the mouth apart and back. The same result can be achieved by placing a thin straw horizontally in the student's mouth.
2. With the mouth stretched, ask the student to say vocalic [r].

Fourth Method (retroflex or bunched) _____

This method works because if a student lies back and relaxes, the tongue "bunches" and falls into the position for vocalic [r]. Though it seems funny, sometimes after establishing vocalic [r] flat on the back, you need to work for the student to say the sound when not reclining.

Objects: None

Instructions: Instruct the student to lie on his or her back, relax the mouth, and say vocalic [r].

Fifth Method (bunched) _____

Objects: None

Instructions:

1. Ask the student to lower the tongue tip.
2. Next, ask the student to hump up the back of the tongue as for "a silent [k]."
3. Ask the student to make the sides of the back of the tongue touch the insides of the back teeth.
4. Lastly, ask the student to turn on the voice box, resulting in vocalic [r].

Shaping Techniques

For many students, it is easier to shape vocalic [r] from another sound than it is to teach it using phonetic placement techniques.

Vocalic (r) (bunched) from (w) _____

This method requires a number of steps, but is effective with the right student.

Objects: Tongue depressor (optional)

Instructions:

1. Lower the student's jaw slightly.
2. Ask the student to say [w].
3. Next, ask the student to make the tongue position for [d].
4. Lastly, ask the student to retract the tongue slightly while lowering the tongue tip and to say vocalic [r].

Vocalic (r) (retroflex) from (n), (d), or (l) _____

This "stretching" technique is very similar to the third vocalic [r] phonetic placement technique.

Objects: Thin drinking straw

Instructions:

1. Ask the student to "make a face" by hooking the first finger of each hand in the corner of the mouth and stretching the mouth apart and back. The same result can be achieved by placing a thin straw horizontally in the student's mouth.
2. With the mouth stretched, ask the student to say a prolonged [n], [d], or [l].
3. As the student says the prolonged [n], [d], or [l], ask him or her to curl the tongue backward, resulting in *ner, der,* or *ler.*
4. Have the student delete the consonant, resulting in vocalic [r].

Vocalic (r) (bunched) from (d) _____

Objects: None

Instructions: Lower the student's jaw slightly as for [d]. While the student's jaw is lowered, ask the student to pull back the tongue slightly, to lower the tongue tip, and to say vocalic [r].

Vocalic (r) (retroflex) from (ð) _____

Objects: None

Instructions:

1. Ask the student to place his or her tongue as for [ð]
2. Ask the student to quickly draw the tongue tip back and slightly up, which typically results in vocalic [r].

Vocalic (r) (retroflex) from Alveolar Trill _____

The trick of this method is to get a student to make an alveolar trill.

Objects: None

Instructions:

1. Instruct the student to trill the tongue tip at the alveolar ridge.
2. Ask the student to stop the trill, but to continue vocalizing, resulting in vocalic [r].

Vocalic (r) (retroflex) from (l) _____

The authors of almost all phonetic placement and shaping techniques are unknown. The exception is the first technique for shaping vocalic [r] from [l], described by Shriberg (1975). The technique works well with a student who can pronounce [l]. The other two techniques offer additional possibilities for shaping [l] into vocalic [r].

First Method (Retroflex)

Objects: None

Instructions:

1. Instruct the student to place the tongue tip on the alveolar ridge in the position for [l].
2. Ask the student to say [l] several times.
3. Ask the student to say [l] for 5 seconds.
4. Next, ask the student to say a long [l], but to drag the tongue tip slowly back along the roof of the mouth until it is so far back that the student has to drop it, resulting in vocalic [r].

Second Method (Retroflex)

Objects: None

Instructions:

1. Ask the student to say [l].
2. While the student says [l], gently pull down the student's jaw until the position for vocalic [r] is reached, resulting in vocalic [r]. (Alternatively, instead of lowering the student's jaw, ask the student to lower his or her jaw).

Third Method (Retroflex)

Objects: Tongue depressor or lollipop stick

Instructions:

1. Ask the student to say [l].
2. Using either a tongue depressor or lollipop stick, gently push back the tongue tip until there is enough space between the tongue tip and roof of the mouth to insert the tongue depressor or lollipop stick, resulting in vocalic [r].

Vocalic (r) (retroflex) from (ʃ)

This clever technique relies on the surprising similarities between vocalic [r] and [ʃ], both of which involve slightly rounded lips, raising of the tongue blade, and contact between the tongue sides and the insides of the teeth. Anne Hommes of Corvalis, Oregon contributed to this technique.

Objects: None

Instructions:

1. Ask the student to say [ʃ], and then ask him or her to turn on the voice box, resulting in [3].
2. Next, ask the student to curl the tongue tip back while keeping contact with the insides of the back teeth, resulting in vocalic [r].

Vocalic (r) from ah

Here are two simple methods for converting ah *into vocalic [r], For both, watch carefully that the student does not round the lips, which results in a vocalic [r] with [w] qualities. If need be, ask the student to hold down the lower lip while practicing.*

First Method (retroflex)

Objects: None

Instructions:

1. Ask the student to sweep the roof of the mouth with the tongue tip while saying ah.
2. Tell the student to stop, but to keep vocalizing *ah*.
3. Instruct the student to lower the tongue tip slightly, which often results in vocalic [r].

Second Method (retroflex)

Objects: None

Instructions:

1. Ask the student to say a long *ahhhhhh*.
2. As the student says *ahhhh*, instruct him or her to raise and curl back the tongue tip, resulting in *ahhhhrrr* (vocalic [r]).

Shell for Speech Exercises

Student's Name: _____

Date: _____

Treatment Sound: _____

Word List: Student Responses:

                                             1. _____

                                             2. _____

                                             3. _____

                                             4. _____

                                             5. _____

                                             6. _____

                                             7. _____

                                             8. _____

                                             9. _____

                                           10. _____

Total Correct: _____ / _____

Comments:

Imitation

Student's Name: _____

Date: _____

Treatment Sound: _____

Goal: Have the student repeat the word after you.

Instructions to Student: "You are going to hear a word with our sound. Please say it after me. Here's an example. I say *sat*, and then you say *sat*."

Word List:	Student Responses:
Sir	1. _____
Dagger	2. _____
Finger	3. _____
Singer	4. _____
Bur	5. _____
Winner	6. _____
Glacier	7. _____
Whisper	8. _____
Fir	9. _____
Author	10. _____

Total Correct: _____/_____

Comments:

Minimal Pairs

Student's Name: _____

Date: _____

Treatment Sound: _____

Goal: Have the student first say the word with the treatment sound, then say the rhyming word, and then say the word with the treatment sound.

Instructions to Student: "You are going to hear a word that begins with our sound. Please say the word, then replace our sound with another sound to make the word have a different meaning, and then say the word with our sound again. Here's an example. I say *seal*. You say *seal*, then change [s] to [w] to make *wheel*, and then say *seal* again. Like this: *Seal. Wheel. Seal.*"

Word List: **Student Responses:**

1. _____

2. _____

3. _____

4. _____

5. _____

6. _____

7. _____

8. _____

9. _____

10. _____

Total Correct: _____ /_____

Comments:

Deletion

Student's Name: _____

Date: _____

Treatment Sound: _____

Goal: Have the student first say the word with the treatment sound, then without the treatment sound, and then with the treatment sound.

Instructions to Student: "You are going to hear a word with our sound. Please say the word, and then say it with our sound deleted, and then say it with our sound included. Here's an example. I say *red*. You say *red*, then *Ed*, then *red*. Like this: *Red. Ed. Red.*"

Word List:		Student Responses:
Singer	sing	1. _____
Winner	win	2. _____
Spider	spied	3. _____
Trailer	trail	4. _____
Steamer	steam	5. _____
Racer	race	6. _____
Chester	chest	7. _____
Cellar	cell	8. _____
Rooster	roost	9. _____
Dancer	dance	10. _____

Total Correct: _____ / _____

Comments:

Self-Correction

Student's Name: _____

Date: _____

Treatment Sound: _____

Goal: Have the student say the word three times, self-correcting if errors in the treatment sound occur.

Instructions to Student: "You are going to hear a word with our sound. Please say the word three times, listening to how you say our sound and changing it to make it correctly if you say it incorrectly. Here's an example. I say *cheese*, and then you say *cheese* three times, listening to how you say our sound and changing it to make it correctly if you say it incorrectly. Like this: *Cheese. Cheese. Cheese.*"

Word List:	Student Responses:
Sir	1. _____
Dagger	2. _____
Finger	3. _____
Singer	4. _____
Bur	5. _____
Winner	6. _____
Glacier	7. _____
Whisper	8. _____
Fir	9. _____
Author	10. _____

Total Correct: _____ / _____

Comments:

Old Way/New Way

Student's Name: _____

Date: _____

Treatment Sound: _____

Goal: Have the student say the word the new way, the old way, and then the new way again.

Instructions to Student: "You are going to hear a word with our sound. Please say the word, then say it the old way you used to say our sound, and then say it the new way you say our sound. Here's an example. I say *thin*. You say *thin*, then **in*, and then *thin*. Like this: *Thin. *in. Thin.*"

Note: Replace * with the way the student used to say the sound.

Word List:	Student Responses:
Sir	1. _____
Dagger	2. _____
Finger	3. _____
Singer	4. _____
Bur	5. _____
Winner	6. _____
Glacier	7. _____
Whisper	8. _____
Fir	9. _____
Author	10. _____

Total Correct: _____ / _____

Comments:

Similar Sound

Student's Name: _____

Date: _____

Treatment Sound: _____

Goal: Have the student first say the word with the treatment sound, then with the most similar sound the student can make, and then with the treatment sound again.

Instructions to Student: "You are going to hear a word with our sound. Please say the word, then replace our sound with _____*, and then say the word with our sound. Here's an example. I say *sun*. You say *sun*, then **un*, and then *sun* again. Like this: *Sun. **un. Sun.*"

Note: Replace * with a sound the student can pronounce that is phonetically similar to the treatment sound.

Word List:	Student Responses:
Sir	1. _____
Dagger	2. _____
Finger	3. _____
Singer	4. _____
Bur	5. _____
Winner	6. _____
Glacier	7. _____
Whisper	8. _____
Fir	9. _____
Author	10. _____

Total Correct: _____ / _____

Comments:

Complete Word List

Vocalic [r]

Open	*Deletions*
Sir	
Dagger	
Finger	
Singer	sing
Bur	
Winner	win
Glacier	
Whisper	
Fir	
Author	
Spider	spied
Barber	
Trailer	trail
Summer	
Steamer	steam
Grocer	
Racer	race
Sister	
Monster	
Chester	chest
Cellar	cell
Rooster	roost
Dancer	dance
Easter	east
Hamster	
Master	mast
Thriller	thrill
Dollar	doll
Endure	
Rider	ride
Spencer	Spence
Caesar	seize
Plaster	
Lobster	
Toaster	toast
Cancer	

Open

Open	Deletions
Freezer	freeze
Satyr	
Fur	
Her	
Over	
Pepper	pep

Closed

Lizard	Burst	Turk
Sneakers	Sure	Curve
Orchard	Pearl	Thunder
Songbird	Girl	Yogurt
Worm	Curb	Self-serve
Bird	Herb	T-shirt
Shirt	Suburb	Work
Burn	Birch	Nerve
Hurl	Church	Girl
Nurse	Bird	Squirrel
Purse	Herd	Germ
Hearse	Leonard	Cavern
Burst	Mustard	Dirt
Thirst	Wizard	Shirt
Burr	Pittsburgh	

Themes for Vocalic [r]

Themes:

Creatures
It's a Job
People to See

Creatures

Creatures	Deletions
Spider	spied
Rooster	roost
Hamster	

Creatures   Deletions

Monster
Lobster
Songbird
Worm
Satyr
Lizard
Squirrel
Bird
Germ

It's a Job   Deletions

Author
Barber   barb
Singer   sing
Racer   race
Dancer   dance
Rider   ride
Wizard
Nurse

People to See   Deletions

Chester   chest
Spencer   Spence
Caesar   seize
Pittsburgh
Turk
Herb
Leonard

References

Shriberg, L. (1975). A response evocation program for vocalic [r]. *Journal of Speech and Hearing Disorders, 40*, 92–105.

Chapter Eight

Consonantal

[r]

Definition

Consonantal [r] (henceforth simply called [r]) is the consonant counter-part of vocalic [r]. [r] occurs before vowels in *read*, *red*, and *three*, and after vowels in *beard*, *hear*, *far*, and *four*. In common with vocalic [r], the consonantal [r] has two variations, the first (bunched) in which the lips are rounded slightly, the tongue tip lowered, and the tongue body bunched up near the area of the palate, and the second (retroflex) in which the lips are rounded slightly and tongue tip is raised to the alveolar ridge or curled back toward the alveolar ridge. In both varieties, the sides of the tongue touch the insides of the teeth about halfway back. As mentioned in the description of vocalic [r], both the bunched and retroflex variations can produce an acceptable [r], though the author's clinical experience is that more students find the bunched variation somewhat easier to learn than the retroflex one.

Acquisition

[r] is acquired by 50% of children by 5;0 and 75% of children by 6;0.

Relative Frequency

[r] is ranked 3rd in relative frequency compared to the other late-acquired consonants. It ranks 8th in relative frequency compared to all other English consonants, and its percentage of occurrence compared to all English consonants is 5.2%.

Errors

The most common error is Gliding—typically, [w] for [r], though [j] also occurs. Deletion of [r] after a vowel and in consonant clusters also is common.

Key Environments

Before a high front vowel, as in **read** [rid]
Between vowels, as in tea_r_y
In a syllable-initial consonant velar cluster, as in **creek**

Possible Metaphors

The metaphors for [r] are the same as for vocalic [r].

[r] quality:	Mad dog or growling tiger sound (grr)
	Arm wrestling sound (errr)
	Pirate sound (aar)
Tongue placement:	Tongue tip flat sound (bunched)
	Tongue tip up sound (retroflex)
Voicing:	Motor on
	Buzzing sound
	Voice box on sound

Touch Cue

The same touch cue is used for [r] as for vocalic [r].

Palm down and finger tips curled down (bunched) or palm up and finger tips curled up (retroflex).

Instructions:

Place the student's hand beside the mouth.

Initial Screening Test for [r]

Student's Name: _____

Date: _____

Referral: _____

Instructions: Say to the student, "I'm going to say some words. Please say the words after me."
Example: "Dog. Now you say it."

Word	Student*	Word	Student*
Beginning			
1. Rain	_____	6. Crayon	_____
2. Root	_____	7. Sprinkle	_____
3. Rat	_____	8. Stream	_____
4. Priest	_____	9. Scream	_____
5. Tribe	_____		
Medial			
10. Story	_____		
11. Gary	_____		
12. Earring	_____		
Final			
13. Oar	_____	16. Airport	_____
14. Stair	_____	17. Starve	_____
15. Spear	_____	18. Mark	_____

Suggestion: Transcribe an X if the sound is correct or, if incorrect, phonetically transcribe the error. Ignore errors produced elsewhere in the word.

Comments/Notes:

Stimulability Tests for [r]

Student's Name: _____

Date: _____

Referral: _____

Imitation

1. rain   _____
2. road   _____

3. bear   _____
4. deer   _____

Best Bet Environments

Before a high front vowel

1. read   _____
2. reek   _____

Between vowels

1. eery   _____
2. teary   _____

In a syllable-initial consonant velar cluster

1. Creek   _____
2. Gray   _____

Favorite Words

Names of family members: _____

Favorite people, heroes, and activities: _____

Phonetic Placement _____

Instruct the student to make a sound like a motor starting up, *rerrrr*.

Shaping (r) from Vocalic (r) _____

1. Ask the student to say vocalic [r] (as in girl).
2. Next, ask the student to say vocalic [r] followed by [i] or some other vowel.
3. Instruct the student to say vocalic [r] + [i] several times as quickly as possible.

Notes/Comments:

Demonstrations for Consonantal [r]

Place: Alveolar

First Method

Object: None

Instructions:

1. Instruct the student, "Please stick out your tongue."
2. Once the tongue is out, for [r] with the tongue tip raised ask the student to pull the tongue back to feel the bump on the roof of the mouth behind the two front teeth. For [r] with the tongue tip down, ask the student to pull the tongue back to feel the little bump behind the two lower teeth.

Second Method

Objects: Q-tip, peanut butter or other favored food

Instructions:

1. Instruct the student, "Please open your mouth."
2. One the mouth is open, with Q-tip dab a little peanut butter or other favorite food on alveolar ridge (for tongue tip raised [r]) or behind lower front teeth (for tongue tip lowered [r]).
3. Ask the student to touch the food with the tongue tip.

Manner: Liquid

First Method

Objects: None

Instructions: Run your or the student's finger down the student's arm while making several long glides or liquids to demonstrate the "flowing" quality and length of this sound.

Second Method

Objects: Strip of paper, a feather, or a small paper flower taped on the end of a pencil

Instructions: Use a strip of paper, a feather, or the hand held in front of the student's mouth while you produce several glides or liquids to draw attention to the "flowing" quality and continuous nature of the sounds. Alternatively, tape a small paper flower on the end of a pencil and encourage the student to move the flower in the wind.

Special Demonstration: Bunched

A Q-tip, small piece of candy, or other favored food sometimes is helpful in demonstrating where to place the tongue tip.

First Method

Objects: None

Instructions: Ask the student to place the tongue tip behind the lower front teeth and to raise the body of the tongue toward the mouth roof.

Second Method

Objects: Q-tip or small piece of candy or other favored food

Instructions:

1. Touch behind the student's lower front teeth with a Q-tip to demonstrate where the tongue tip should be placed. Alternatively, place a small piece of candy or other favored food behind the lower front teeth and ask the student to hold it there with the tongue tip.
2. Once this is achieved, ask the student to raise the tongue body toward the mouth roof.

Special Demonstration: Retroflex

A Q-tip, small piece of candy, or other favored food sometimes is helpful in demonstrating where to place the tongue tip.

Method

Objects: None

Instructions:

1. Ask the student to place the tongue tip behind the upper front teeth.
2. Ask the student to curl the tongue backward without touching the roof of the mouth until it cannot go back farther.

Sides of Tongue (Bunched and Retroflex): Vocalic and Consonantal [r]

A good [r] often is more easily achieved if the student is encouraged to say the sound while keeping the sides of the tongue touching the insides of the teeth. The following simple demonstration can be practiced in isolation or as part of the bunched and retroflex demonstrations.

First Method

Objects: None

Instructions:

1. Tell the student that his or her tongue is sleepy and wants to rest.
2. Instruct the student to let the tongue spread out in "its bed" until it is touching the insides of the teeth.

Second Method

Objects: Q-tip, candy, or other favored food

Instructions:

1. Touch the inside teeth with a Q-tip or some favored food to demonstrate where the tongue should go.
2. Tell the student that his or her tongue is sleepy and wants to rest.
3. Instruct the student to let the tongue spread out in "its bed" until it is touching the insides of the teeth.

Voicing: Voiced

First Method

Objects: None

Instructions: Instruct the student to listen to and identify the difference between a voiceless and voiced [a].

Second Method

Objects: None

Instructions: Place the student's hands over the ears and instruct him or her to hum, which heightens the sensation of vocal cord vibration.

Third Method

Objects: None

Instructions: If the student is able to produce a voiced and voiceless fricative, ask him or her to cover the ears and make these sounds. Alternatively, the student is asked to make [h] and [a].

Fourth Method

Objects: None

Instructions: You and the student place one hand on your throat and the other on the student's throat while making voiced and voiceless sounds together, telling each other when the voicing goes on and off.

Fifth Method

Objects: Pencil, small piece of paper or small paper flower

Instructions: If the student is able to produce a voiced and voiceless oral stop, attach a small piece of paper or a paper flower to the end of a tongue depressor or pencil and ask the student to "make the paper (or flower) move." The paper is more likely to move when a voiceless consonant is produced than when a voiced consonant is produced (be careful in providing instructions to the student, however, because a strongly articulated voiced oral stop will also move the flower).

Phonetic Placement and Shaping Techniques for [r]

Phonetic Placement Techniques

First Method

Objects: None

Instructions: Ask the student to make a sound like a motor starting up (ruh).

Second Method

Objects: Tongue depressor (optional)

Instructions:

1. Ask the student to place the tongue tip behind the upper front teeth. (If needed, place the student's tongue tip on a shelf made with a tongue depressor.)
2. Next, ask the student to curl the tongue backward without touching the roof of the mouth until it cannot go back farther.
3. Lower the student's jaw slightly and ask the student to say [ru].

Shaping Techniques

(r) from vocalic (r)

These two methods are for a student who has mastered vocalic [r]. They are the methods the author uses most often to teach [r].

First Method

Objects: None

Instructions:

1. Ask the student to say vocalic [r].
2. Next, ask the student to say vocalic [r] before a word beginning with [r]. For example, say *read* as vocalic [r] + [rid].

3. After the student pronounces the words with vocalic [r] followed by consonantal [r], instruct him or her to say the vocalic [r] silently, which typically results in initial [r].

Second Method

This method relies on the fact that a syllable that ends in vocalic [r] and is followed by a syllable beginning with a vowel will often result in a syllable-initial [r] as a type of transition between vocalic [r] and the vowel that follows.

Objects: None

Instructions:

1. Ask the student to say vocalic [r].
2. Next, ask the student to say vocalic [r] followed by [i] or some other vowel.
3. Instruct the student to say vocalic [r] + [i] several times as quickly as possible, resulting in vocalic [r] − [ri]. After [ri] is established, instruct the student to say vocalic [r] silently. The resulting sound is [ri].

(r) from (w)

This method is for a student who substitutes [w] for [r] (Gliding), but whose tongue is in the correct position for [r]. Such a student may need to be taught to reduce lip rounding.

Objects: Tongue depressor (optional)

Instructions:

1. Lower the student's jaw slightly.
2. Ask the student to say [w] but to "let the lips go to sleep" or "make it with a little smile." An alternative method is to tell the student, "No kissing frogs" to prompt an unround lip position. If needed, gently push the student's lips back with a tongue depressor to an unrounded lip position.

(r) from (a)

This and the following method are for students for whom you wish to establish [r] at the end of syllables. The methods demonstrate the technique for [ar] as in car and [ir] as in bear. The same technique works for all other vowels. To illustrate, to teach [or] as in simply replace [a] or [i] with [o]. When teaching [r] in this position, a useful trick is to have the student keep contact between the sides of the tongue and the inner teeth.

Objects: None

Instructions:

1. Ask the student to say *ah*.
2. Next, ask the student to raise the tongue slightly toward the roof of the mouth and say [ɑr]. (If needed, instruct the student to raise the tongue tip or to raise the tongue slightly and to say [a] forcibly.) The resulting sound is [ɑr].

(r) from (i) _____

Objects: None

Instructions:

1. Ask the student to say [i].
2. While the student says [i], ask him or her to lift the tongue and curl back the tongue tip to say [ir].

Shell for Speech Exercises

Student's Name: _____

Date: _____

Treatment Sound: _____

Word List: Student Responses:

                                    1. _____

                                    2. _____

                                    3. _____

                                    4. _____

                                    5. _____

                                    6. _____

                                    7. _____

                                    8. _____

                                    9. _____

                                    10. _____

Total Correct: _____/_____

Comments:

Imitation

Student's Name: _____

Date: _____

Treatment Sound: _____

Goal: Have the student repeat the word after you.

Instructions to Student: "You are going to hear a word with our sound. Please say it after me. Here's an example. I say *sat*, and then you say *sat*."

Word List:

Rain

Root

Relaxed

Rat

Rattle

Robot

Rug

Rainy

Red Sea

Raven

Student Responses:

1. _____

2. _____

3. _____

4. _____

5. _____

6. _____

7. _____

8. _____

9. _____

10. _____

Total Correct: _____ / _____

Comments:

Minimal Pairs

Student's Name: _____

Date: _____

Treatment Sound: _____

Goal: Have the student first say the word with the treatment sound, then say the rhyming word, and then say the word with the treatment sound.

Instructions to Student: "You are going to hear a word that begins with our sound. Please say the word, then replace our sound with another sound to make the word have a different meaning, and then say the word with our sound again. Here's an example. I say *seal*. You say *seal*, then change [s] to [w] to make *wheel*, and then say seal again. Like this: *Seal. Wheel. Seal.*"

Word List:

Rat	sat
Rug	bug
Root	toot
Rattle	saddle
Reach	beach
Read	bead
Rocks	socks
Roast	toast
Run	sun
Rink	sink

Student Responses:

1. _____
2. _____
3. _____
4. _____
5. _____
6. _____
7. _____
8. _____
9. _____
10. _____

Total Correct: _____ / _____

Comments:

Deletion

Student's Name: _____

Date: _____

Treatment Sound: _____

Goal: Have the student first say the word with the treatment sound, then without the treatment sound, and then with the treatment sound.

Instructions to Student: "You are going to hear a word with our sound. Please say the word, and then say it with our sound deleted, and then say it with our sound included. Here's an example. I say *red*. You say *red*, then *Ed*, then *red*. Like this: *Red. Ed. Red.*"

Word List:		Student Responses:
Rat	at	1. _____
Rattle	addle	2. _____
Read	Ed	3. _____
Rocks	ox	4. _____
Rhino	I know	5. _____
Red	Ed	6. _____
Reach	each	7. _____
Rose	owes	8. _____
Rita	eat a	9. _____
Rome	om	10. _____

Total Correct: _____ / _____

Comments:

Self-Correction

Student's Name: _____

Date: _____

Treatment Sound: _____

Goal: Have the student say the word three times, self-correcting if errors in the treatment sound occur.

Instructions to Student: "You are going to hear a word with our sound. Please say the word three times, listening to how you say our sound and changing it to make it correctly if you say it incorrectly. Here's an example. I say *cheese*, and then you say *cheese* three times, listening to how you say our sound and changing it to make it correctly if you say it incorrectly. Like this: *Cheese. Cheese. Cheese.*"

Word List:	Student Responses:
Rain	1. _____
Root	2. _____
Relaxed	3. _____
Rat	4. _____
Rattle	5. _____
Robot	6. _____
Rug	7. _____
Rainy	8. _____
Red Sea	9. _____
Raven	10. _____

Total Correct: _____ / _____

Comments:

Old Way/New Way

Student's Name: _____

Date: _____

Treatment Sound: _____

Goal: Have the student say the word the new way, the old way, and then the new way again.

Instructions to Student: "You are going to hear a word with our sound. Please say the word, then say it the old way you used to say our sound, and then say it the new way you say our sound. Here's an example. I say *thin*. You say *thin*, then **in*, and then *thin*. Like this: *Thin. *in. Thin.*"

Note: Replace * with the way the student used to say the sound.

Word List: **Student Responses:**

Rain   1. _____

Root   2. _____

Relaxed   3. _____

Rat   4. _____

Rattle   5. _____

Robot   6. _____

Rug   7. _____

Rainy   8. _____

Red Sea   9. _____

Raven   10. _____

Total Correct: _____ / _____

Comments:

Similar Sound

Student's Name: _____

Date: _____

Treatment Sound: _____

Goal: Have the student first say the word with the treatment sound, then with the most similar sound the student can make, and then with the treatment sound again.

Instructions to Student: "You are going to hear a word with our sound. Please say the word, then replace our sound with _____*, and then say the word with our sound. Here's an example. I say *sun*. You say *sun*, then *un*, and then *sun* again. Like this: *Sun. *un. Sun.*"

Note: Replace * with a sound the student can pronounce that is phonetically similar to the treatment sound.

Word List:	Student Responses:
Rain	1. _____
Root	2. _____
Relaxed	3. _____
Rat	4. _____
Rattle	5. _____
Robot	6. _____
Rug	7. _____
Rainy	8. _____
Red Sea	9. _____
Raven	10. _____

Total Correct: _____/_____

Comments:

Complete Word List for Consonantal [r]

Beginning of Words

Single Consonants	Deletions	Minimal Pairs
Rain		vein, mane, pane, pain
Root		toot, moot
Relaxed		
Rat	at	sat, mat, bat, pat, fat, hat, cat
Rattle	addle	saddle, battle, cattle
Robot		
Rug		bug, mug, jug, hug
Rainy		
Red Sea		
Raven		cave-in, maven
Read	Ed	bead, seed, weed
Rabbit		habit
Roast		toast, coast, most
Rocks	ox	socks, box, fox
Rhino	I know	
Red	Ed	bed, wed, head
Reach	each	beach, teach, leech
Rowboat		
Russia		
Rose	owes	toes, mows
Richard		
Reptile		
Railroad		
Ring		sing, wing, king
Rita	eat a	pita
Rome	om	home, gnome
Raccoon		
Rice	ice	mice, nice
Rope		soap, hope
Row	owe	mow, no, know, sow, go
Rugby		
Run		sun, bun, one, gun, fun
Rachel		
Road	ode, owed	toad, mowed
Rink	ink	sink, wink, pink, link
Room		tomb

Single Consonants	Deletions	Minimal Pairs
Wrestle		trestle
Ron	on	gone
Roof		goof
Rainbow		
Realm	elm	helm
Rake	ache	bake, make, lake, shake
Race	ace	face, chase, lace
Reef		leaf
Ruth		
Rust		dust, bust
Ram	am	Sam, Pam, lamb
Raisin		lazin'
Rod	odd	mod, sod, nod, god
Roll		bowl, goal
Raincoat		
Roar	oar, or	tore, soar
Rip		whip, lip, hip
Rinse		mince
Racket		
Write		night, light, fight
Ran	an	can, man, pan
Reel	eel	kneel, feel, deal, Neal
Robed		
Ripe		pipe, type
Rail	ale	nail, whale, mail, jail, veil, tail, pail
Rind		mind, signed, bind
Roy	Oi	boy, toy
Ray		bay, say, May
Ranch		
Rip		tip, lip, whip, ship
Rag		bag, sag, nag
Rebel		
Raid	aid	maid, jade
Rhine		mine, fine, sign
Rend	end	bend, send, mend
Ramon		
Rake	ache	bake, take, lake
Rich	itch	witch, hitch

Consonant Clusters	Deletions

(pr)

Prize	pies
Price	
Prince	
Preschool	
Preach	peach
Prairie	Perry
Prowl	Powell
Pray	pay
Proof	poof
Prison	
Press	
Princess	
Prune	
Priest	pieced
Prick	pick
Pretzel	
Pray	pay
Pro	

(tr)

Trip	tip
Track	tack
Train	
Trent	tent
Tractor	
Tree	tea, T
Trunk	
Tray	
Travel	
Tribe	
Tragic	
Trick	tick
Tramp	
Traffic	
Trap	tap
Trail	tail
Trash can	
Truck	tuck
Troll	toll

Consonant Clusters   *Deletions*

Tree house
Trouble
Treat   teat
Trailer   tailor
Trash
Tracy
Trish   Tish

(kr)

Crab   cab
Crib
Cradle
Crown
Crawl
Crayon
Crumbs   comes
Crow
Crash   cash
Cricket
Crete
Christmas
Chris   kiss
Croak   coke
Creak
Crossbow
Crutch
Crust   cussed
Crisp
Cry

(br)

Bread   bed
Broom   boom
Brownie
Brian
Braces   bases
Britain
Brick   Bic
Broken
Bridge

Consonant Clusters	Deletions
Branch	
Brake	bake
Broomstick	
Brazil	
Brain	bane
Bronze Age	
Brush	
Break	bake

(dr)

Drink	dink
Driftwood	
Drive	dive
Driver	diver
Drill	dill
Dry	die
Drugstore	
Drag race	
Dragon	
Drum	dumb
Drawer	
Driveway	
Drag	
Dreaming	deeming
Drip	dip
Drizzle	
Dress	
Drain	Dane
Drummer	dumber

(gr)

Grass	gas
Grease	geese
Great	gate
Grapefruit	
Grant	
Grave	gave
Grover	
Grizzly	
Group	

Consonant Clusters	**Deletions**
Grouchy	
Grapes	gapes
Ground	
Greece	geese
Great Dane	
Gray	gay
Green	
Grow	go
Grill	gill
Grocer	

(fr)

Front	
Frown	
Fruit	
French fries	
Friday	
Fry	fie
Francis	
Frank	
Freeze	fees
Franklin	
Frog	fog
Frosting	
Friend	fend
Friar	fire
France	

(θr)

Three	thee
Throw	though
Thrill	
Throttle	
Thrift shop	
Thread	
Throat	
Threw	
Throw rug	
Thriller	

Consonant Clusters	Deletions
Throne	
Thrifty	
Throwing	
Threshold	
Throng	thong
Thrive	
Thrash	
Through	
Thrush	
Threat	
Thrust	
Throb	

(ʃr)

Shrew	rue
Shredded	
Shrug	rug
Shrimp	
Shrub	rub
Shroud	
Shreveport	
Shrivel	
Shriek	reek
Shred	red
Shrill	rill
Shrink	rink
Shrine	Rhine
Shrewd	rude

(spr)

Spring	
Spray	spay
Sprite (soda)	spite
Sprinkles	
Spray gun	
Spruce	
Spry	spy
Sprint	
Sprinkle	
Springboard	

Consonant Clusters   *Deletions*

Sprinkling
Springtime
Sprain   Spain
Sprinkler
Spread   sped
Spring
Sprig
Spree
Spruce
Sprout
Sprawl

(str)

Struck   stuck
Strum
Strike out
Strong
Stroller
Street
Stranger
Straw
Stronghold
Stripe
String   sting
Strike zone
Streetcar
Stream   steam
Strap
Strike
Stretcher
Strict   sticked
Stroke   stoke
Struggle
Strut

(skr)

Screen
Scribble
Scream   scheme
Scratch

Consonant Clusters	Deletions
Scrapper	
Scrooge	
Screenplay	
Scrub	
Screw	
Script	skipped
Scramble	
Scribe	
Scrap	
Scroll	
Scrimp	skimp
Scrabble	
Screech	

Consonant + (r)	Deletions
Britain	
Prize	pies
Trap	tap
Price	
Prince	
Throat	
Preschool	
Bridge	
Prairie	Perry
Frosting	
Prowl	
Pray	pay
Grease	geese
Prison	
Trouble	
Priest	pieced
Trip	tip
Crayon	
Travel	
Drummer	dumber
Tribe	
Drip	dip
Trick	tick
Prune	
Tramp	

Consonant + (r)   *Deletions*

Traffic	
Grow	go
Truck	tuck
Frog	fog
Troll	toll
Driver	diver
Trailer	tailor
Trish	Tish
Crib	
Trash can	
Crown	
Prick	pick
Crawl	
Thrill	
Crow	
Track	tack
Crash	cash
Drugstore	
Cricket	
Trail	tail
Crete	
Dress	
Croak	coke
Friar	fire
Creak	
Tree house	
Crutch	
Preach	peach
Crust	cussed
Princess	
Crisp	
Bronze Age	
Cry	
Bread	bed
Tracy	
Brownie	
Tree	tea, T
Brian	
Tragic	
Brake	bake
Green	
Broomstick	

Consonant + (r)	Deletions
Crumbs	comes
Brazil	
Crab	cab
Brain	bane
Shriveled	
Brush	
Pro	
Break	bake
Train	
Crossbow	
Trunk	
Press	
Tray	
Drink	
Friday	
Driftwood	
Throttle	
Drive	dive
Broken	
Drill	dill
Christmas	
Dry	die
Brick	
Drag race	
Friend	fend
Drawer	
Driveway	
Trash	
Drag	
Tractor	
Drizzle	
Broom	boom
Drain	Dane
Grass	gas
Prof	
Great	gate
Grapefruit	
Grant	
French fries	
Grave	gave
Freeze	fees
Grizzly	

Consonant + (r)   Deletions

Consonant + (r)	Deletions
Group	
Grouchy	
Drum	dumb
Grapes	gapes
Braces	bases
Gray	gay
Shroud	
Grill	gill
Branch	
Grocer	
Front	
Frown	
Pray	pay
Fruit	
Dreaming	deeming
Fry	fie
Trent	tent
Francis	
Chris	kiss
Frank	
Thriller	
Franklin	
France	
Three	
Shriek	sheik
Throw	
Thrush	
Cradle	
Thread	
Dragon	
Throw rug	
Grover	
Thrum	thumb
Greece	geese
Thrift shop	
Shrimp	
Pretzel	
Shrub	
Great Dane	
Shrew	shoe
Ground	
Shrink	

Consonant + Consonant + (r)   *Deletions*

Scribe	
Spring	
Scrooge	
Strike out	
Sprint	
Sprawl	
String bean	
Sprinkle	
Stream	steam
Scream	scheme
Straight	state
Spray	spay
Straw	stall
Sprinkler	
Strut	
Spry	spy
Scrawny	
Sprinkling	
Stride	
Sprig	
Street	
Spruce	
Stretcher	
Springboard	
Strudel	
Stripe	
Spread	sped
Strap	
Scratchy	
Spree	
Stretch	
Scribble	
Strange	
Scrub	
Stroller	
Sprinkles	
Screw	
Springtime	
Strong	
Scrapbook	
Spray gun	

Consonant + Consonant + (r)   Deletions

String	sting
Sprout	
Screech	
Sprain	Spain
Scratch	
Sprite	spite

Medial

Single Consonants

Story	Garage	Tourist
Gary	Berry	Beret
Earring	Forest	Syringe
Marry	Laura	Eric
Barrel	Zero	Arrow
Europe	Merry	Peru
Harry	Sheriff	Cairo
Arrest	Burro	Ferry
Irish	Weary	Sarah
Zorro	Very	Terry
Hero	Carol	Far East

Consonant Clusters

(pr)

Surprise	Apron	Depressed
Supreme	Blueprint	Cypress
Footprint	Soundproof	
Shipwreck	April	

(tr)

Country	Portrait	Mattress
Subtract	Actress	Pine tree
Pantry	Waitress	Subtract
Fire truck	Race track	Entrance
Matrix	Detroit	Patrick

Consonant Clusters

(kr)

Secret	Concrete	King crab
Aircraft	Witchcraft	Akron
Across	Red Cross	Pie crust
Red Crescent	Recruit	Cock roach
Scarecrow	Spacecraft	

(br)

Umbrella	Toothbrush	Hairbrush
Fabric	Hebrew	Zebra
Cornbread	Library	Cambridge

(dr)

Laundry	Gum drop	Hydrant
Address	Bedroom	Ear drop
Hundred	Madrid	Raindrop
Children	Soft drink	

(gr)

Regret	Pilgrim	School grounds
Hungry	Bridegroom	Background
Agree	Photograph	
Congress	Angry	

(fr)

Defrost	Deep freeze	French fries
Afraid	Bull frog	Grapefruit
Cold front	Boyfriend	

(ðr)

Bathrobe	Drive through	Heart throb

(ʃr)

Mushroom	Washrag	Washroom

Consonant Clusters

(spr)

Hot springs	Hair spray
Bedspread	Offspring

(str)

Bloodstream	Shoestring	High-strung
Construct	Backstroke	Nostril
Monstrous	Nostril	Pastry

(skr)

Ice cream	Corkscrew	Subscribe
Describe	Muskrat	

All Consonant Clusters

Subscribe	Ear drop	Soft drink
Portrait	Witchcraft	Akron
Subtract	Fire truck	Regret
Construct	Red Cross	Hungry
Surprise	Afraid	Hundred
Depressed	Recruit	Agree
Cypress	Pie crust	Spacecraft
Country	Gum drop	Congress
Cold front	Bloodstream	Deep freeze
Monstrous	Cockroach	Pilgrim
Entrance	Umbrella	Bedspread
Patrick	Corkscrew	Bridegroom
Secret	Fabric	April
Blueprint	Hydrant	Photograph
Muskrat	Cornbread	Hot springs
Aircraft	Address	School grounds
Raindrop	Toothbrush	Children
Across	Hebrew	Background
Red Crescent	Pantry	Apron
Shipwreck	Defrost	Angry
Scarecrow	Bedroom	Bull frog
Matrix	Hairbrush	Library
Concrete	Madrid	Boyfriend

All Consonant Clusters

King crab
Subtract
French fries
Supreme
Grapefruit
Bathrobe
Actress
Waitress
Race track
Drive through
Cambridge

Heart throb
Mushroom
Footprint
Washrag
Zebra
Laundry
Washroom
Detroit
Hair spray
Offspring
Soundproof

Shoestring
Backstroke
Mattress
Nostril
High-strung
Nostril
Pastry
Ice cream
Pine tree
Describe

All Environments

Subscribe
Portrait
Weary
Subtract
Construct
Surprise
Depressed
Cypress
Country
Garage
Zero
Cold front
Monstrous
Entrance
Story
Gary
Earring
Irish
Patrick
Secret
Very
Blueprint
Muskrat
Berry
Aircraft
Raindrop
Across

Red Crescent
Shipwreck
Carol
Scarecrow
Matrix
Marry
Barrel
Concrete
Ear drop
Witchcraft
Fire truck
Red Cross
Tourist
Afraid
Recruit
Pie crust
Gum drop
Laura
Bloodstream
Cockroach
Umbrella
Arrest
Corkscrew
Fabric
Hydrant
Cornbread
Europe

Address
Toothbrush
Hebrew
Forest
Pantry
Defrost
Bedroom
Beret
Hairbrush
Madrid
Soft drink
Akron
Harry
Regret
Syringe
Hungry
Hundred
Agree
Hero
Spacecraft
Congress
Arrow
Deep freeze
Pilgrim
Bedspread
Bridegroom
April

All Environments

Photograph
Hot springs
School grounds
Eric
Children
Background
Apron
Angry
Bull frog
Library
Peru
Boyfriend
King crab
Subtract
French fries
Supreme
Merry
Grapefruit

Bathrobe
Actress
Waitress
Zorro
Race track
Drive through
Cambridge
Cairo
Heart throb
Mushroom
Sarah
Footprint
Washrag
Zebra
Far East
Laundry
Washroom
Detroit

Sheriff
Hair spray
Offspring
Ferry
Soundproof
Shoestring
Terry
Backstroke
Mattress
Nostril
High-strung
Burro
Nostril
Pastry
Ice cream
Pine tree
Describe

End of Words

End of Words*

*Deletions are not included for [r] at the end of words. The [r] lowers the preceding vowel, making the deletions task for this sound less useful for most students.

Car
Guitar
Oar
Stair
Spear
Door
Poor
Jar
Seashore
Tear
Year
Bazaar
Bar
Ore
Pier

End of Words *

Software
Soar
Share
Hear
Ear
Space bar
Bookstore
Pour
Air
Snack bar
Stare
Frontier
War
Pear
Nightmare
Cheer
New Year
Star
Scar
Swear
Scare
North Star
Chair
Downpour
Steer
Senor
Mare
Shore
Air
Bear
Boar
Square
Hair
Éclair
Four
Floor
Boar
Store

Consonant Clusters   *Deletions*

(rt)

Art
Airport
Court
Port
Head Start
Heart
Tart
Starve

(rk)

Arc
Mark
Bark
Pitchfork
Denmark
Ark
Dark
New York
Pork
Fork

(rb)

Rhubarb
Barb

(rd)

Beard
Blackboard
Lord
Flashcard
Hard
Bored
Hoard
Award

Consonant Clusters   Deletions

(rg)

Morgue
Borg

(rm)

Arm
Farm
Storm
Snowstorm

(rn)

Born
Corn
Horn
Thorn
Torn
Popcorn
Acorn

(rs)

Horse

(rʃ)

Borsch

(rtʃ)

Arch
March
Porch
Starch
Torch
Research

Consonant Clusters   Deletions

(rd)

Barge
Large
Forge
George

(r) + consonant

Snowstorm
Art
Denmark
Airport
Starve
Mark
George
Acorn
Bark
Torn
Pitchfork
Farm
Dark
Popcorn
Fork
Rhubarb
Port
Beard
Pork
Blackboard
Borg
Lord
Barb
Flashcard
Court
Hard
Tart
Bored
Arc
Hoard
New York
Award
Morgue

Consonant Clusters   Deletions

Arm
Porch
Storm
Born
Forge
Horn
Torch
Thorn
Horse
Borsch
Arch
Heart
March
Corn
Starch
Research
Barge
Ark
Large
Head Start

Themes for Consonantal [r]

Themes:

Around the Home	Halloween Stories
Food	People to See
Animals	Places to Go
Scary Noises	

Around the Home	Deletions	Minimal Pairs
Rug	ugh	bug, mug, jug, hug
Trash		
Floor	flow	
Chair		
Stair		
Rake	ache	bake, take, lake
Rag		bag, sag, nag
Garage		

Around the Home	**Deletions**	**Minimal Pairs**
Roof		goof
Room		tomb
Door		
Broom	boom	

Food	**Deletions**	**Minimal Pairs**
Roast		toast, most, coast
Sprinkles		
Strudel		
String bean		
Rice	ice	mice, nice
Rich	itch	witch, hitch
Fruit		
French fries		
Pear		
Frosting		
Snack bar		
Éclair		
Prune		
Sprite	spite	
Cornbread		
Raisin		lazin'
Pretzel		
Crab	cab	
Crumbs	comes	
Crust	cussed	
Bread	bed	
Brownie		
Grapefruit		
Grapes	gapes	
Shrimp		
King crab		
Pie crust		
Gum drop		
Soft drink		
Pastry	pasty	
Mushroom		
Ice cream		
Popcorn		
Corn		

Food	**Deletions**	**Minimal Pairs**
Rhubarb		
Pork		
Tart		
Borsch		

Animals	**Deletions**	**Minimal Pairs**
Rat	at	sat, mat, bat, pat, fat, hat, cat
Dragon		
Burro		
Raven		cave-in, maven
Rabbit		habit
Rhino		
Reptile		
Frog	fog	
Raccoon		
Ram	am	Sam, Pam, lamb
Great Dane		
Shrew		
Cockroach		
Crow		
Roar	oar	tore, soar, more, boar
Steer		
Mare	May	
Bear	bay	
Boar		
Grizzly		
Shrimp		
Bull frog		
Muskrat		
Horse		
Zebra		
Cricket		

Scary Noises	**Deletions**	**Minimal Pairs**
Hear	he	
Ear	E	
Croak	coke	
Creak		

Scary Noises	*Deletions*	*Minimal Pairs*
Crash	cash	
Scratchy		
Screech		
Shriek	sheik	
Drip	dip	
Cry		
Bark		
Roar	oar	tore, soar, more, boar

Halloween Stories	*Deletions*	*Minimal Pairs*
Trick	tick	
Treat	teat	
Hoard	hoed	
Heart		
Rend	end	bend, send, mend
Afraid		
Witchcraft		
Strange		
Shroud		
Shriveled		
Thriller		
Thrill		
Friar	fire	
Grave	gave	
Dreaming		
Broomstick		
Crossbow		
Crown		
Tree	tea, T	
Trunk		
Princess		
Scare		
Nightmare		
Spear		
Arrow		
Forest		
Hero		
Ring		sing, wing, king
Rain		vein, mane, pane, pain
Story		

Halloween Stories	Deletions	Minimal Pairs
Rainy		
Downpour		
Hair	hay, hey	
Priest	pieced	
Secret		
Children		
Dark		
Morgue		
Storm		
Thorn		
Torch		

People to See	Deletions	Minimal Pairs
Rose	owes	toes, mows
Richard		
Rita	eat a	pita
Rachel		
Ron	on	
Ruth		
Rod	odd	mod, sod, nod, god
Roy	Oi	boy, toy
Ramon		
Ray	A	bay, say, May
Gary		
Harry		
Zorro		
Laura		
Sarah		
Terry		
Carol		
Eric		
Tracy		
Trish	Tish	
Brian		
Patrick		
April		
Scrooge		
Franklin		
Grover		
Francis		

People to See	*Deletions*	*Minimal Pairs*
Frank		
George		
Barb	Bob	
Mark		
Chris	kiss	

Places to Go	*Deletions*	*Minimal Pairs*
Red Sea		
Russia		
Rome	om	home, gnome, roam
Europe		
Far East		
Peru		
Cairo		
North Star		
Rhine		mine, fine, sign
Crete		
Brazil		
Britain		
Detroit		
Greece	geese	
France		
(The) Matrix		
Akron		
New York		
Denmark		
Madrid		

Chapter Nine

[ʃ]

Definition

[ʃ] is made behind the alveolar ridge, a little behind the position for [s]. The tongue blade is raised, and the lips are rounded. The airstream is continuous and the vocal folds are apart. The technical definition of [ʃ] is voiceless postalveolar fricative.

Acquisition

[ʃ] is acquired by 50% of children by 3;6 and by 75% of children by 5;0.

Relative Frequency

[ʃ] is ranked 6th in relative frequency compared to the other late-acquired consonants. It ranks 19th in relative frequency compared to all other English consonants, and its percentage of occurrence compared to all English consonants is 1.5%.

Errors

[s] for [ʃ] is a common error. A younger student may pronounce [ʃ] as [t] or [d]. A less common, though not rare error, is pronouncing [ʃ] as [tʃ].

Key Environments

End of a syllable or word, as in *fish*
Before a high front vowel, as in *she*

Possible Metaphors

The best metaphors for [ʃ] typically focus on the fricative nature of the sound.

Tongue placement:	Back of the hill sound
Fricative:	Hushing sound
	Shhh! sound
	Quiet sound
	Long sound
Voicing:	Motor on
	Buzzing sound
	Voice box on sound

Touch Cue

Finger in front of lips and use the metaphor "quiet sound."

Instruction:

Place the student's finger in the corner of the lips, and remind the student that this is the quiet sound.

Initial Screening Test for [ʃ]

Student's Name: _____

Date: _____

Referral: _____

Instructions: Say to the student, "I'm going to say some words. Please say the words after me."
Example: "Dog. Now you say it."

Word   **Student***

Beginning

  1. Shell   _____

  2. Shutter   _____

  3. Show   _____

  4. Shrug   _____

  5. Shrimp   _____

  6. Shred   _____

Medial

  7. Wishing   _____

  8. Ocean   _____

  9. Washer   _____

Final

10. Dish   _____

11. Crush   _____

12. Irish   _____

13. Harsh   _____

14. Marsh   _____

15. Borsch   _____

***Suggestion:** Transcribe an X if the sound is correct or, if incorrect, phonetically transcribe the error. Ignore errors produced elsewhere in the word.

Comments/Notes:

Stimulability Tests for [ʃ]

Student's Name: _____

Date: _____

Referral: _____

Imitation

1. **sh**oe   _____
2. bu**sh**   _____

Best Bet Environments

End of a syllable or word

1. fi**sh**   _____
2. [i**sh**]   _____

Before a high front vowel

1. **sh**e   _____
2. **sh**y   _____

Favorite Words

Names of family members: _____

Favorite people, heroes, and activities: _____

Phonetic Placement _____

1. Ask the student to hiss like a snake.
2. While the student hisses, ask him or her to purse the lips.

Shaping (ʃ) from (s) _____

1. Ask the student to say [s].
2. Instruct him or her to pucker the lips slightly and to draw the tongue back a little until [ʃ] results.

Notes/Comments:

Demonstrations for [ʃ]

Place: Postalveolar

First Method

Objects: None

Instructions: Ask the student to run the tongue to where the bump on the mouth roof just begins to go down toward the back of the mouth, using an analogy of a "hill and valley."

Second Method

Objects: Q-tip, peanut butter or other favored food

Instructions:

1. Instruct the student, "Please open your mouth."
2. Once the mouth is open, with Q-tip dab a little peanut butter or other favorite food behind the alveolar ridge.
3. Ask the student to touch the food with the tongue blade.

Manner: Fricative

First Method

Objects: Strip of paper or a feather

Instructions:

1. Place a strip of paper, a feather, or the student's hand held in front of your mouth while you produce several long voiceless fricatives.
2. Draw attention to the "hissing" quality and continuous nature of the sounds.

Second Method

Objects: A small paper flower on end of a pencil

Instructions: Tape a small paper flower on the end of a pencil and encourage the student to move the flower in the wind.

Third Method

Object: None

Instructions: Run your finger or the student's finger down the student's arm while making several long voiceless fricatives to demonstrate the "hissing" quality and length of fricatives.

Voicing: Voiceless

First Method

Objects: None

Instructions: Instruct the student to listen to and identify the difference between a voiceless and voiced [a].

Second Method

Objects: None

Instructions: Place the student's hands over the ears and instruct him or her to hum, which heightens the sensation of vocal cord vibration.

Third Method

Objects: None

Instructions: If the student is able to produce a voiced and voiceless fricative, ask him or her to cover the ears and make these sounds. Alternatively, the student is asked to make [h] and [a].

Fourth Method

Objects: None

Instructions: You and the student place one hand on your throat and the other on the student's throat while making voiced and voiceless sounds together, telling each other when the voicing goes on and off.

Fifth Method

Objects: Pencil, small piece of paper or small paper flower

Instructions: If the student is able to produce a voiced and voiceless oral stop, attach a small piece of paper or a paper flower to the end of a tongue depressor or pencil and ask the student to "make the paper (or flower) move." The paper is more likely to move when a voiceless consonant is produced than when a voiced consonant is produced (be careful in providing instructions to the student, however, because a strongly articulated voiced oral stop will also move the flower).

Phonetic Placement and Shaping Techniques for [ʃ]

Phonetic Placement Technique

Method

In this book there is only a single phonetic placement exercise for [ʃ]. Most often, the sound is easily established through a demonstration or a shaping exercise.

Objects: Tongue depressor (optional)

Instructions:

1. Ask the student to part the teeth and lips.
2. Touch the student's tongue just behind the tip with a tongue depressor. Ask the student to move the place just touched to the roof of the mouth behind the "bumpy part." (If needed, a tongue depressor may be used to push the tongue back from the upper front teeth.)
3. Next, ask the student to lower the tongue slightly. (If needed, direct the tongue down slightly with a tongue depressor.)
4. Ask the student to hold this position, pucker the lips slightly, and breathe out through the mouth, resulting in [ʃ].

Shaping Techniques

(ʃ) from (s)

This is a good, efficient method for a student with a well-established [s].

Object: None

Instructions: Ask the student to say [s]. While the student is saying [s], instruct him or her to pucker the lips slightly and to draw the tongue back a little until [ʃ] results.

(ʃ) from (ʒ)

Most students do not have a well-established [ʒ] before having a well-established [ʃ]. For those who do, however, this method works well.

Objects: None

Instructions: Ask the student to say [ɜ] and then turn off the voice, which often results in [ʃ].

(ʃ) from (i)

As for the [ʃ] from [i] shaping technique, this technique relies on the fact that [ʃ] and [i] are made near the same place of production.

Objects: None

Instructions:
1. Ask the student to say [i], first with the voice on and then with the voice off.
2. Next, ask the student to pucker the lips slightly.
3. Raise the student's lower jaw slightly.
4. Ask the student to breathe out silently while raising the tongue. The sound produced is [ʃ].

Shell for Speech Exercises

Student's Name: _____

Date: _____

Treatment Sound: _____

Word List: Student Responses:

                                              1. _____

                                              2. _____

                                              3. _____

                                              4. _____

                                              5. _____

                                              6. _____

                                              7. _____

                                              8. _____

                                              9. _____

                                            10. _____

Total Correct: _____ / _____

Comments:

Imitation

Student's Name: _____

Date: _____

Treatment Sound: _____

Goal: Have the student repeat the word after you.

Instructions to Student: "You are going to hear a word with our sound. Please say it after me. Here's an example. I say *sat*, and then you say *sat*."

Word List:	**Student Responses:**
Shoe	1. _____
Sheep	2. _____
Shiny	3. _____
Shut	4. _____
Sharon	5. _____
Shovel	6. _____
Shell	7. _____
Shutter	8. _____
Show	9. _____
Shannon	10. _____

Total Correct: _____ / _____

Comments:

Minimal Pairs

Student's Name: _____

Date: _____

Treatment Sound: _____

Goal: Have the student first say the word with the treatment sound, then say the rhyming word, and then say the word with the treatment sound.

Instructions to Student: "You are going to hear a word that begins with our sound. Please say the word, then replace our sound with another sound to make the word have a different meaning, and then say the word with our sound again. Here's an example. I say *seal*. You say *seal*, then change [s] to [w] to make *wheel*, and then say *seal* again. Like this: *Seal. Wheel. Seal.*"

Word List:		Student Responses:
Shoe	goo	1. _____
Ship	chip	2. _____
Sheet	feet	3. _____
Show	row	4. _____
Shoe	two	5. _____
Shake	lake	6. _____
Shy	hi	7. _____
Shore	tore	8. _____
Shear	tear	9. _____
Shock	knock	10. _____

Total Correct: _____ / _____

Comments:

Deletion

Student's Name: _____

Date: _____

Treatment Sound: _____

Goal: Have the student first say the word with the treatment sound, then without the treatment sound, and then with the treatment sound.

Instructions to Student: "You are going to hear a word with our sound. Please say the word, and then say it with our sound deleted, and then say it with our sound included. Here's an example. I say *red*. You say *red*, then *Ed*, then *red*. Like this: *Red. Ed. Red.*"

Word List: **Student Responses:**

Shoe	uh	1. _____
Sharon	Aaron	2. _____
Shell	L	3. _____
Shutter	utter	4. _____
Show	o, owe	5. _____
Sheet	eat	6. _____
Shade	aid	7. _____
Shy	I, eye	8. _____
Sheik	eek	9. _____
Shower	hour	10. _____

Total Correct: _____/_____

Comments:

Self-Correction

Student's Name: _____

Date: _____

Treatment Sound: _____

Goal: Have the student say the word three times, self-correcting if errors in the treatment sound occur.

Instructions to Student: "You are going to hear a word with our sound. Please say the word three times, listening to how you say our sound and changing it to make it correctly if you say it incorrectly. Here's an example. I say *cheese*, and then you say *cheese* three times, listening to how you say our sound and changing it to make it correctly if you say it incorrectly. Like this: *Cheese. Cheese. Cheese.*"

Word List:	Student Responses:
Shoe	1. _____
Sheep	2. _____
Shiny	3. _____
Shut	4. _____
Sharon	5. _____
Shovel	6. _____
Shell	7. _____
Shutter	8. _____
Show	9. _____
Shannon	10. _____

Total Correct: _____ /_____

Comments:

Old Way/New Way

Student's Name: _____

Date: _____

Treatment Sound: _____

Goal: Have the student say the word the new way, the old way, and then the new way again.

Instructions to Student: "You are going to hear a word with our sound. Please say the word, then say it the old way you used to say our sound, and then say it the new way you say our sound. Here's an example. I say *thin*. You say *thin*, then **in*, and then *thin*. Like this: *Thin. *in. Thin.*"

Note: Replace * with the way the student used to say the sound.

Word List:	**Student Responses:**
Shoe	1. _____
Sheep	2. _____
Shiny	3. _____
Shut	4. _____
Sharon	5. _____
Shovel	6. _____
Shell	7. _____
Shutter	8. _____
Show	9. _____
Shannon	10. _____

Total Correct: _____ / _____

Comments:

Similar Sound

Student's Name: _____

Date: _____

Treatment Sound: _____

Goal: Have the student first say the word with the treatment sound, then with the most similar sound the student can make, and then with the treatment sound again.

Instructions to Student: "You are going to hear a word with our sound. Please say the word, then replace our sound with _____*, and then say the word with our sound. Here's an example. I say *sun*. You say *sun*, then **un*, and then *sun* again. Like this: *Sun. *un. Sun.*"

Note: Replace * with a sound the student can pronounce that is phonetically similar to the treatment sound.

Word List:	Student Responses:
Shoe	1. _____
Sheep	2. _____
Shiny	3. _____
Shut	4. _____
Sharon	5. _____
Shovel	6. _____
Shell	7. _____
Shutter	8. _____
Show	9. _____
Shannon	10. _____

Total Correct: _____ / _____

Comments:

Complete Word List for [ʃ]

Beginning of Words

Single Consonants	Deletions	Minimal Pairs
Shoe	oo	goo, boo, new, dew, Sue
Sheep		cheep, keep, peep, jeep, deep, leap
Shiny		
Shut		mutt, gut
Sharon	Aaron	
Shovel		hovel
Shell	L	bell, fell
Shutter	utter	gutter, butter
Show	o, owe	bow, go, toe, mow
Shannon		cannon
Sheet	eat	feet, meat, neat, beet, beat
Shade	aid	paid, raid, wade
Shortcake		
Shield		field, kneeled
Sugar		bugger
Cheryl		barrel, Carol
Shock		knock, rock, sock, lock
Shy	I, eye	hi, lie, die, buy, cry
Shellfish		
Shine		vine, sign, nine, line
Sherlock		
Sheik	eek	beak, meek, seek, peek
Shower	hour	tower, power, cower
Shortcut		
Shaw	awe	law, saw
Shed	Ed	dead, said, wed, head
Shout	out	pout
Shady		
Shane		pain, sane, bane, mane
Sherbet		
Shamrock		
Shore	or, ore	tore, more, core, chore
Shoelace		
Shortbread		
Shadow		

Single Consonants	*Deletions*	*Minimal Pairs*
Shirt		hurt, dirt
Shepherd		
Shape	ape	cape, nape, tape
Shakespeare		
Shark	arc, ark	dark, bark, lark
Sheriff		
Ship		chip, sip, hip, zip, whip, rip, lip
Shampoo		
Shush		hush, mush
Shake	ache	lake, bake, make, rake
Short		court
Shaft	aft	raft, laughed
Shuffle		ruffle
Shoe	oo	two, new, boo, dew
Shadow		
Shear	ear	tear, near, beer, seer
Shop		hop, pop, mop
Sharp		tarp, carp
Sham	aim	came, tame, same
Shed	Ed	bed, Ned, red
Shaggy	Aggie	baggy
Shift		gift, lift
Shave		pave, knave
Shanty		ante
Shiver		liver, giver
Shade	aid	laid, maid, paid
Shelter		
Shabby	abbey	cabbie, tabby
Shape		tape, nape
Shot		hot, got, pot, rot
Shock		rock, sock, knock
Shaking	aching	baking, making
Shower	hour	power, tower, bower
Shoulder	older	colder, bolder
Shelob		
Shale	ail, ale	mail, nail, pail, tail
Shallow	aloe	callow, tallow
Shelf	elf	
Sham	am	ram, Pam, Sam, ham
Show	O	row, tow, mow, go
Share	air, heir	care, mare, tear
Shuttle		

Consonant Clusters	**Deletions**	**Minimal Pairs**
Shrew	rue	grew, true, brew
Shredded		breaded
Shrug	rug	drug
Shrimp		crimp
Shrub	rub	grub
Shroud		crowd
Shreveport		
Shrug	rug	
Shrivel		drivel
Shriek	reek	creek
Shred	red	tread, bread
Shrill	rill	trill, krill
Shrink	rink	brink
Shrine	Rhine	
Shrewd	rude	crewed, brewed

Medial

Single Consonants

Wishing	Washcloth	Woodshed
Ocean	Bushes	Fractions
Washer	Dishes	Flash card
Banshee	Windshield	Nashville
Fishing	Ashes	Dishcloth
Rickshaw	Flashlight	Push-ups
Sunshine	Dashboard	Seashore
Glacier	Snowshoe	Washtub
Handshake	Washing	
Fishy	Steamship	

Consonant Clusters

—

End of Words

Single Consonants	*Deletions*
Mustache	
Trash	
Dash	
Goldfish	
Irish	
Dish	
Crush	
British	
Crawfish	
Mash	
Crash	
Toothbrush	
Fish	
Cash	
Catfish	
Hush	
Spanish	
Ash	
Wash	
Welsh	well
Paintbrush	
Leash	Lee
Clash	
Trish	
Push	
Nailbrush	
Flush	
Wish	
Splash	
Car wash	
Bush	
Josh	
Rubbish	
Smash	
Danish	
Mouthwash	

Consonant Clusters	Deletions
Harsh	
Marsh	mar
Borsch	bore

Themes for [ʃ]

Themes:

People to See	Watery Places
Places to Go	Things to Eat
Creatures	Washing Dishes
Things That Go Bump in the Night	

People to See	Deletions	Minimal Pairs
Sharon		
Shannon		cannon
Cheryl		barrel, Carol
Sherlock		
Shaw	awe	
Shane		cane, bane, mane
Shakespeare		
Irish		
Ash		
Wash		
Welsh	well	
Spanish		
British		
Shaggy	Aggie	baggy
Shelob		
Trish		
Josh		
Danish		

Places to Go	Deletions	Minimal Pairs
Nashville		
Shreveport		

Creatures	Deletions	Minimal Pairs
Sheep		cheep, keep, peep, jeep, deep, leap
Shark		dark, bark, lark
Goldfish		
Fish		
Crawfish		
Catfish		
Shrew	rue	true, brew, grew
Shrimp		

Things That Go Bump	Deletions	Minimal Pairs
Banshee		
Shelob		
Shape		tape, nape
Shiver		liver, giver
Shade	aid	laid, maid, paid
Sharp		tarp, carp
Shadow		
Shock		rock, sock, knock
Shaking	aching	baking, making
Shrivel		drivel
Shriek	reek	creek

Watery Places	Deletions	Minimal Pairs
Shale	ail, ale	mail, nail, pail, tail
Shallow	aloe	callow, tallow
Ocean		
Fishing		
Seashore		
Shelf	elf	
fishy		
Shark		dark, bark, lark
Shore	or, ore	tore, more, core, chore
Ship		chip, sip, hip, zip, whip, rip, lip
Splash		
Shell	L	bell, fell
Goldfish		
Shower	hour	power, tower, bower

Watery Places	**Deletions**	**Minimal Pairs**
Fish		
Crawfish		
Catfish		
Shrimp		
Steamship		

Things to Eat	**Deletions**	**Minimal Pairs**
Shortcake		
Sugar		
Shellfish		
Fish		
Crawfish		
Catfish		
Shrimp		
Shake	ache	lake, bake, make, rake
Sherbet		
Shortbread		
Borsch	bore	

Washing Dishes	**Deletions**	**Minimal Pairs**
Dish		
Rubbish		
Splash		
Trash		
Dishes		
Washcloth		
Washing		
Washer		
Shine		vine, sign, nine, line

Chapter Ten

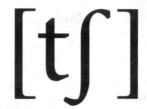

Definition

[tʃ] is made with the body of the tongue touching the mouth roof behind the bumpy ridge (alveolar ridge). The lips are slightly puckered. The airstream is stopped and then becomes continuous, making it a short stop ([t]) followed by a fricative ([tʃ]). The vocal folds are apart. The technical definition of [tʃ] is voiceless postalveolar affricate.

Acquisition

[tʃ] is acquired by 50% of children by 4;6 and by 75% of children by 5;6.

Relative Frequency

[tʃ] is ranked 8th in relative frequency compared to the other late-acquired consonants. It ranks 22nd in relative frequency compared to all other English consonants, and its percentage of occurrence compared to all English consonants is 0.7%.

Errors

Errors for [tʃ] typically keep either the stop or fricative component of the sound. Both [t] for [tʃ] and [s] for [ʃ] are common.

Key Environments

End of a syllable or word, as in *batch*
After a high front vowel, as in *witch*

Possible Metaphors

The best metaphors for [tʃ] typically focus on the affricate (stop-fricative) quality of the sound.

Affricate quality: Choo-choo sound
                         Sneezing sound (choo!)
                         Engine-chugging sound

Tongue placement: Back of the hill sound

Voicing: Motor on
                         Buzzing sound
                         Voice box on sound

Touch Cue

None.

Initial Screening Test for [tʃ]

Student's Name: _____

Date: _____

Referral: _____

Instructions: Say to the student, "I'm going to say some words. Please say the words after me."
Example: "Dog. Now you say it."

Word	Student*
Beginning	
1. Chain	_____
2. Chip	_____
3. Chunk	_____
Medial	
4. Peaches	_____
5. Itchy	_____
6. Teacher	_____
Final	
7. Witch	_____
8. Sketch	_____
9. Itch	_____
10. Porch	_____
11. Starch	_____
12. Punch	_____

Suggestion: Transcribe an X if the sound is correct or, if incorrect, phonetically transcribe the error. Ignore errors produced elsewhere in the word.

Comments/Notes:

Stimulability Tests for [tʃ]

Student's Name: _____

Date: _____

Referral: _____

Imitation

   1. **ch**ip   _____

   2. cat**ch**   _____

Best Bet Environments

End of a syllable or word

   1. [Itʃ]   _____

   2. wat**ch**   _____

After a high front vowel

   1. bea**ch**   _____

   2. it**ch**   _____

Favorite Words

Names of family members: _____

Favorite people, heroes, and activities: _____

Phonetic Placement _____

   1. Ask the student to make the train sound, "choo choo."

Shaping _____

   1. Instruct student to say "Bet you" slowly.

   2. Next, instruct student to say "Bet you" fast, resulting in the production of "Betcha."

   3. If "betcha" doesn't work, repeat with "Got you."

Notes/Comments:

Demonstrations for [tʃ]

Place: Postalveolar

First Method _____

Objects: None

Instructions: Ask the student to run the tongue to where the bump on the mouth roof just begins to go down toward the back of the mouth, using an analogy of a "hill and valley."

Second Method _____

Objects: Q-tip, peanut butter or other favored food

Instructions:

1. Instruct the student, "Please open your mouth."
2. Once the mouth is open, with Q-tip dab a little peanut butter or other favorite food behind the alveolar ridge.
3. Ask the student to touch the food with the tongue blade.

Manner: Affricate

Method _____

Objects: None

Instructions: Have the student hold his or her hands together tightly and then separate them quickly to indicate the stop onset and fricative release of affricates.

Voicing: Voiceless

First Method _____

Objects: None

Instructions: Instruct the student to listen to and identify the difference between a voiceless and voiced [a].

Second Method

Objects: None

Instructions: Place the student's hands over the ears and instruct him or her to hum, which heightens the sensation of vocal cord vibration.

Third Method

Objects: None

Instructions: If the student is able to produce a voiced and voiceless fricative, ask him or her to cover the ears and make these sounds. Alternatively, the student is asked to make [h] and [a].

Fourth Method

Objects: None

Instructions: You and the student place one hand on your throat and the other on the student's throat while making voiced and voiceless sounds together, telling each other when the voicing goes on and off.

Fifth Method

Objects: Pencil, small piece of paper or small paper flower

Instructions: If the student is able to produce a voiced and voiceless oral stop, attach a small piece of paper or a paper flower to the end of a tongue depressor or pencil and ask the student to "make the paper (or flower) move." The paper is more likely to move when a voiceless consonant is produced than when a voiced consonant is produced (be careful in providing instructions to the student, however, because a strongly articulated voiced oral stop will also move the flower).

Phonetic Placement and Shaping Techniques for [tʃ]

Phonetic Placement Technique

Method

Objects: None

Instructions:

1. Ask the student to pucker the lips slightly.
2. Ask the student to make the tongue tip touch "the bump" behind the two upper front teeth.
3. Next, instruct the student to make the sneezing sound (choo!) while keeping the lips slightly puckered and the tongue tip on the alveolar ridge. If [ts] results, ask the student to move the tongue tip back slightly while maintaining contact with the roof of the mouth. The resulting sound is [tʃ].

Shaping Technique

(tʃ) from (ʃ)

Objects: None

Instructions: Ask the student to say a quick [ʃ] with the tongue tip touching "the bump," resulting in [tʃ]. (*Note:* To facilitate [dʒ], develop from [ʒ].)

(tʃ) from (t) and (ʃ)

Objects: None

Instructions:

1. Explain that [tʃ] is [t] and [ʃ] said together very quickly.
2. Next, ask the student to say [ʃ].
3. Instruct the student to say [t] and then to draw the tongue tip back a little and say [t] again.
4. With the student's tongue tip in the position for the "back" [t], instruct the student to quickly say [t] followed by [ʃ], which typically results in [tʃ]. (*Note:* To facilitate [dʒ], develop from [d] and [dʒ].)

(tʃ) from (ts)

*This method modifies [ts] as in **pizza** into [tʃ]*

Objects: None

Instructions:

1. Instruct the student to say *pizza*.
2. Next, ask the student to say only the [ts] in *pizza*. (If needed, have the student divide *pizza* into two parts—pi-zza—and then ask the student to say only the second part—zza.
3. Next, ask the student to say [ts] farther back in the mouth, resulting in [tʃ].

Shell for Speech Exercises

Student's Name: _____

Date: _____

Treatment Sound: _____

Word List: Student Responses:

                                         1. _____

                                          2. _____

                                          3. _____

                                          4. _____

                                          5. _____

                                          6. _____

                                          7. _____

                                          8. _____

                                          9. _____

                                        10. _____

Total Correct: _____/_____

Comments:

Imitation

Student's Name: _____

Date: _____

Treatment Sound: _____

Goal: Have the student repeat the word after you.

Instructions to Student: "You are going to hear a word with our sound. Please say it after me. Here's an example. I say *sat*, and then you say *sat*."

Word List:	Student Responses:
Cheese	1. _____
Chicken	2. _____
Chief	3. _____
Cheat	4. _____
Chain	5. _____
Chip	6. _____
Chunk	7. _____
Church	8. _____
Chuck	9. _____
Chop	10. _____

Total Correct: _____ / _____

Comments:

Minimal Pairs

Student's Name: _____

Date: _____

Treatment Sound: _____

Goal: Have the student first say the word with the treatment sound, then say the rhyming word, and then say the word with the treatment sound.

Instructions to Student: "You are going to hear a word that begins with our sound. Please say the word, then replace our sound with another sound to make the word have a different meaning, and then say the word with our sound again. Here's an example. I say *seal*. You say *seal*, then change [s] to [w] to make *wheel*, and then say seal again. Like this: *Seal. Wheel. Seal.*"

Word List: **Student Responses:**

Chore	boar	1. _____
Chill	pill	2. _____
Charge	barge	3. _____
Chunk	skunk	4. _____
Cheese	peas	5. _____
Cheep	sheep	6. _____
Chum	mum	7. _____
Chop	shop	8. _____
Chest	test	9. _____
Cheer	fear	10. _____

Total Correct: _____ / _____

Comments:

Deletion

Student's Name: _____

Date: _____

Treatment Sound: _____

Goal: Have the student first say the word with the treatment sound, then without the treatment sound, and then with the treatment sound.

Instructions to Student: "You are going to hear a word with our sound. Please say the word, and then say it with our sound deleted, and then say it with our sound included. Here's an example. I say *red*. You say *red*, then *Ed*, then *red*. Like this: *Red. Ed. Red.*"

Word List:		Student Responses:
Cheese	ease	1. _____
Cheat	eat	2. _____
Chew	oo	3. _____
Chase	ace	4. _____
Chin	in	5. _____
Cheek	eek	6. _____
Chicks	icks	7. _____
Chess	s	8. _____
Chill	ill	9. _____
Cherry	airy	10. _____

Total Correct: _____ / _____

Comments:

Self-Correction

Student's Name: _____

Date: _____

Treatment Sound: _____

Goal: Have the student say the word three times, self-correcting if errors in the treatment sound occur.

Instructions to Student: "You are going to hear a word with our sound. Please say the word three times, listening to how you say our sound and changing it to make it correctly if you say it incorrectly. Here's an example. I say *cheese*, and then you say *cheese* three times, listening to how you say our sound and changing it to make it correctly if you say it incorrectly. Like this: *Cheese. Cheese. Cheese.*"

Word List:	Student Responses:
Cheese	1. _____
Chicken	2. _____
Chief	3. _____
Cheat	4. _____
Chain	5. _____
Chip	6. _____
Chunk	7. _____
Church	8. _____
Chuck	9. _____
Chop	10. _____

Total Correct: _____ / _____

Comments:

Old Way/New Way

Student's Name: _____

Date: _____

Treatment Sound: _____

Goal: Have the student say the word the new way, the old way, and then the new way again.

Instructions to Student: "You are going to hear a word with our sound. Please say the word, then say it the old way you used to say our sound, and then say it the new way you say our sound. Here's an example. I say *thin*. You say *thin*, then **in*, and then *thin*. Like this: *Thin. *in. Thin.*"

Note: Replace * with the way the student used to say the sound.

Word List: **Student Responses:**

Cheese   1. _____

Chicken   2. _____

Chief   3. _____

Cheat   4. _____

Chain   5. _____

Chip   6. _____

Chunk   7. _____

Church   8. _____

Chuck   9. _____

Chop   10. _____

Total Correct: _____ / _____

Comments:

Similar Sound

Student's Name: _____

Date: _____

Treatment Sound: _____

Goal: Have the student first say the word with the treatment sound, then with the most similar sound the student can make, and then with the treatment sound again.

Instructions to Student: "You are going to hear a word with our sound. Please say the word, then replace our sound with _____*, and then say the word with our sound. Here's an example. I say *sun*. You say *sun*, then **un*, and then *sun* again. Like this: *Sun. *un. Sun.*"

Note: Replace * with a sound the student can pronounce that is phonetically similar to the treatment sound.

Word List:	Student Responses:
Cheese	1. _____
Chicken	2. _____
Chief	3. _____
Cheat	4. _____
Chain	5. _____
Chip	6. _____
Chunk	7. _____
Church	8. _____
Chuck	9. _____
Chop	10. _____

Total Correct: _____/_____

Comments:

Complete Word List for [tʃ]

Beginning of Words

Single Consonants	Deletions	Minimal Pairs
Cheese	ease	peas, keys, knees
Chicken		sicken
Chief		thief, beef, leaf
Cheat	eat	seat, meat, heat, wheat
Chain		Spain, gain, lane, pain
Chip		ship, hip, sip, rip, lip, whip, zip, dip
Chunk		skunk, junk
Church		
Chuck		luck, buck, tuck
Chop		shop, cop, pop, top, hop, mop
Chew	oo	zoo, moo, two, shoe, new, boo
Chase	ace	pace, race, case
Chapter		raptor
Charge		barge, large, Marge
Chirp		
Chin	in	pin, thin
Checkers		
Charles		
Cheek	eek	peek, seek, week, leak
Cheetah		
Chicks	eek	six, mix
Chess	S	Wes, mess, less
Chill	ill	pill, gill, Bill, mill
Chest		test, pest, vest, nest, west
Cherry	airy	Sherry, merry, berry
Chilly		Willy, Billy, hilly
Champ	amp	ramp, lamp, damp
Chalk		balk, talk
Chick	ick	lick, sick, wick
Child		tiled, piled
Chili		Willy, Billy, hilly
Cheer	ear	fear, hear, deer, near, year
Cheep		sheep, jeep, deep, leap
Choke	oak	soak, poke
Chair	air	mare, care, fair, hair

Single Consonants	Deletions	Minimal Pairs
China		
Choice		
Chad	add	mad, sad, bad, cad
Chore	ore, or	boar, core, more, tore
Chafe		safe
Cheat	eat	beat, meet, seat
Chatter		matter, tatter, batter
Chain mail		
Chat	at	cat, rat, mat, pat
Chug		bug, hug, mug
Chair	air	tear, wear, care
Choose	ooze	news, lose
Charcoal		
Challenge		
Chamber		
Cherish		perish
Chum	um	mum, hum, sum, come
Chief		beef
Chopstick		
Chance		dance
Champagne		
Church		
Check		peck, neck
Change		mange, range
Channel		panel
Chant	ant	can't, rant, pant
Chap		tap, map, cap
Chapel	apple	
Charm	arm	harm
Checkers		
Charter		barter, martyr
Churn	earn	burn, turn
Chase	ace	face, case, pace
Cheap		peep, keep, deep

Consonant Clusters

None

Medial

Single Consonants

Peaches	Stitches	Nature
Itchy	Future	Pitcher
Rachel	Nachos	Ketchup
Richard	Rancher	Vulture
Picture	Inches	Pitching
Teacher	Roaches	Watching
Matches	Preacher	Benches
Witches	Gretchen	Preacher
Pitchfork	Question	Torture

Consonant Clusters

Archway	Lunchtime	Lunches
Torchlight	Parchment	
Lunchroom	Finches	

All Environments

Archway	Pitchfork	Lunchtime
Peaches	Stitches	Pitcher
Itchy	Future	Ketchup
Finches	Nachos	Vulture
Rachel	Lunchroom	Pitching
Richard	Rancher	Parchment
Picture	Inches	Watching
Torchlight	Roaches	Benches
Teacher	Preacher	Preacher
Matches	Gretchen	Torture
Witches	Question	
Lunches	Nature	

End of Words

Single Consonants   ## Deletions

Teach	tea, T
Witch	

Single Consonants	Deletions
Peach	pea, P
Sketch	
Roach	row
Coach	
Ouch	ow
Speech	
Track coach	
Watch	
Ski coach	
Wristwatch	
Beach	bee, B
Catch	
Couch	cow
Sandwich	
Watch	
Cockroach	
Scratch	
Ostrich	
Fetch	

Consonant Clusters	Deletions

(rtʃ)

Arch	R
Scorch	score
March	mar
Porch	poor, pour
Starch	star

(ntʃ)

Trench	
Punch	pun
Branch	
French	
Bunch	bun
Lunch	
Bench	Ben
Wrench	wren

Themes for [tʃ]

Themes:

Actions   It's a Job
Around the Home   People and Places
The Body   Lunch
Nature

Actions	Deletions	Minimal Pairs
Cheat	eat	seat, meat, heat, wheat
Chased	aced	paste, taste, raced, waist
Sketch		
Watch		
Teach	tea, T	
Catch		
Fetch		
Scratch		
March	mar	
Matches		
Pitching		
Watching		
Choke	oak	soak, poke
Cheer	ear	fear, hear, deer, near, year
Chain		Spain, gain, lane, pain
Charge		barge, large, Marge
Chirp		peek, seek, week, leak
Chip		ship, hip, sip, rip, lip, whip, zip, dip
Chop		shop, cop, pop, top, hop, mop
Chew	oo	zoo, moo, two, shoe
Chill	ill	pill, gill, Bill, mill
Scorch	score	
Choose	ooze	news, lose
Check		peck, neck
Change		mange, range
Chant	ant	can't, rant, pant
Chase	ace	face, case, pace
Chat	at	cat, rat, mat, pat
Cheat	eat	beat, meet, seat
Chatter		matter, tatter, batter
Charm	arm	harm

Around the Home	*Deletions*	*Minimal Pairs*
Porch	pour, poor	
Starch	star	
Arch	R	
Archway		
Couch	cow	
Wrench	wren	
Watch		
Wristwatch		
Picture		
Checkers		
Chess		Wes, mess, less
Chalk		balk, talk
Chopstick		
Chair	air	mare, tear, wear, care
Chore	ore, or	boar, core, more, tore

The Body	*Deletions*	*Minimal Pairs*
Chin	in	pin, thin
Chest		test, pest, vest, nest, west
Cheek	eek	leak, beak, meek

Nature	*Deletions*	*Minimal Pairs*
Roach	row	
Cockroach		
Ostrich		
Branch		
Roaches		
Nature		
Vulture		
Beach	bee, B	
Itchy		
Cheetah		
Chicks		six, mix
Cherry	airy	Sherry, merry, scary

It's a Job | Deletions | Minimal Pairs

Preacher
Teacher
Ski coach
Rancher
Track coach
Coach

People and Places | Deletions | Minimal Pairs

Chuck		luck, buck, tuck
Gretchen		
Rachel		
Richard		
China		
Charles		

Lunch | Deletions | Minimal Pairs

Peaches		
Lunch		
Chew	oo	zoo, moo, two, shoe
Chill	ill	pill, gill, Bill, mill
Lunchtime		
Chip		ship, hip, sip, rip, lip, whip, zip, dip
Scorch	score	
Lunchroom		
Cheese	ease	peas, keys, knees
Chicken		sicken
Chili		hilly, Willy, Billy
Nachos		
Ketchup		
Chop		shop, cop, pop, top, hop, mop
Sandwich		
Punch	pun	
Bunch	bun	
Peaches		
Peach	pea, P	
Cherry	airy	Sherry, merry, scary
Pitcher		
Lunches		

Chapter Eleven

Language Therapy for Speech Disorders

Introduction

Resources in this book may be used in diverse ways within many different approaches. This chapter illustrates how they are employed to evaluate and treat students in one school setting. The illustration is descriptive rather than prescriptive, suggesting how the resources *might* be used rather than indicating how they *should* be used.

Clinical Orientation

Use of resources described in this chapter is based on three ideas:

1. Treatment of late-acquired sounds reflects the dual nature of speech.
2. Treatment success depends as much on human variables as linguistics ones.
3. Treatment activities are functional.

The Dual Nature of Speech

Speech has a dual nature: it is both a channel of communication and a part of language (Bleile, 2004). The dual nature of speech is the basis of the conceptual distinction between an articulation disorder (disorder arising in the channel of communication) and a phonologic disorder (a disorder in the language component).

Articulation

A primary reason the eight are acquired late is that they are hard to pronounce. What late-acquired sounds share in common is that none are made with the articulators touching throughout (as stop consonants and nasals are) or with the articulators relatively far apart (as glides and vowels are). Instead, late-acquired sounds require a student to position the articulators not touching, not far apart, but somewhere in the middle, making the airflow variously stop and start (affricates), hiss (fricatives), flow over the sides of the tongue (lateral), or flow around and over an atypical tongue configuration ([r]). Examples of resources focusing primarily on the articulation aspect of speech include definitions, metaphors, demonstrations, phonetic placement and shaping techniques, and key environments.

Phonology

Being a skilled motor movement is only one-half of speech's dual nature. Speech also is an aspect of language, requiring language knowledge similar to but distinct from knowledge that underlies syntax, morphology, semantics, and discourse. A critical aspect of treating late-acquired sounds entails drawing a student's attention to the communication value of speech. In addition to learning how to pronounce a sound, a student must also learn how sound affects meaning, how a sound is similar to and different from other sounds, and how to self-monitor and self-correct to ensure that communication occurs. Examples of resources focusing primarily on the phonologic aspect of speech include speech exercises, language activities, and word lists.

Human Variables

A speech problem does not exist independently from the person who has the problem. Factors such as motivation, intelligence, family support, attention, and desire to learn are equally important for clinical success as linguistic ones. To give just one illustration of the diversity of the people attached to speech problems, one recent morning three students in the same grade and school received speech therapy, one after the other. The first was embarrassed by his speech problem, the second thought his speech problem sounded pretty cool, and the third didn't know he had a speech problem. Later that same day another student was treated—a teenager with a severe [r] difficulty who desperately wanted speech help for an upcoming radio presentation with his class. He promised to do anything to have better speech—except give up basketball practice for speech therapy. Radio address or not, basketball had a higher priority. The point is not to criticize this priority—only to emphasize that students bring far more than their linguistic system to the therapy setting. Examples of resources focusing primarily on human variables arising in the treatment of late-acquired sounds include acquisition, relative frequencies, and errors.

> ### *Human Variables*
>
> What is more trite and less controversial than the assertion that treatment success depends as much on human variables as linguistic ones? Nonetheless, considering that most clinicians believe such variables are important, it is amazing how poor our knowledge base is about human variables compared to our knowledge of linguistic factors. Far more research is needed before we understand how learner attributes interact with speech factors to influence treatment outcome.

Functional Activities

All students, children, and adults, gifted or delayed, learn and grow throughout their life. Time devoted to treatment of late-acquired sounds should further this learning whenever possible. In practice, this entails using activities that encourage learning and personal growth. Class materials, books, and projects are excellent sources of activities for school-aged students, as newspapers and movies and upcoming social events are for older school-aged students and adults. In addition to providing support for learning, a critical benefit of treatment relying on such activities is that it encourages use of a treatment sound in contexts that matter to a student. Examples of resources that most directly support classroom and life-based activities are the speech exercises and language activities.

Clinical Resources

The order in which resources are described in the following sections is modified slightly from that in Chapter One to better approximate their use with a hypothetical student from the evaluation through conclusion of treatment. The sequence is indicated in Table 11–1.

Evaluation

The following resources are used primarily in assessment:

- Initial Screening
- Screening for stimulability
- Definition
- Acquisition
- Relative frequency
- Errors

Table 11-1. Clinic Resources Used in Evaluation and Treatment.

Assessment	Initial screening
	Screening for stimulability
	Definition
	Acquisition
	Relative frequency
	Errors
Treatment	Metaphors
	Touch cues
	Demonstrations
	Phonetic placement and shaping techniques
	Key environments
	Word lists
	Speech and awareness exercises
	Language activities

Initial Screening, Screening for Stimulability

The most typical referral source for a student is a parent or teacher. A student may then be observed in a classroom or playground before receiving an initial speech screening and a screening test for stimulability.

Initial Screening

An initial screening helps determine if a student experiences difficulty pronouncing a late-acquired sound. An initial screening assesses a treatment sound at the word level in a variety of phonetic contexts. In addition to determining if a problem with a sound exists, an initial screening often serves as a pretest against which treatment progress is measured. If a student's speech is found to contain speech errors, a screening test for stimulability typically is administered.

Screening for Stimulability

Screening for stimulability helps determine if a student can pronounce a possible treatment sound. Information on stimulability is helpful in predicting how rapidly treatment is likely to proceed. In general, if a student has some initial capacity to pronounce a sound, treatment proceeds more rapidly than if such a capacity must first be established.

Definition, Acquisition, Relative Frequency, and Errors

These resources bundle together after stimulability testing is completed and as a clinician decides between possible treatment sounds. Typically, deciding which sound to select is based on weighing multiple factors, personal and linguistic. Personal factors include a clinician's judgment about a student's attention span, interests, and concerns. The linguistic aspect of sound selection includes stimulability, definition, acquisition, relative frequency, and errors. No single variable trumps the others. Rather, a clinician weighs multiple considerations to reach a balanced decision.

Definition

The definition is a prose description showing how a sound is produced. The definition contributes to treatment decisions because understanding how a sound is made suggests which resources may be needed to teach it. To illustrate, for [l] a clinician thinks about where the tongue is, how easily it might be to teach a student this tongue position, what types of demonstrations might be needed, what phonetic placement and shaping technique to use, and the types of exercises available. Alternately, for [s] an additional consideration might be to develop short probes to determine which [s] is easier for a student—tongue tip raised or lowered? Typically, a clinician follows the student's lead—that is, if a student already makes [s] with the tongue tip lowered, the clinician teaches [s] with a lowered tongue. If a student does not have a preferred way, a clinician may feel freer to select an appropriate variant.

Acquisition

Acquisition data indicate the age at which 50% and 75% of children acquire a sound. If all other things are equal (they seldom are), a clinician may decide to first treat an earlier acquired sound. Indeed, for some clinicians the importance of acquisition data is the primary criterion used in the selection process.

Relative Frequency

Relative frequency is the frequency of occurrence of a sound. Typically, remediation of a sound with a higher frequency of occurrence has greater impact on intelligibility than one with lower frequency. For this reason, a clinician may incline to first teach more frequently occurring treatment sounds. To illustrate, if a clinician is deciding between [s] and [z], [s] might be selected because of its higher frequency of occurrence.

Errors

Errors are the major errors to which a sound is susceptible. This information weighs in sound selection in at least two respects:

1. Some errors may be socially stigmatized.
2. Errors have varying effect on intelligibility.

In general, errors that may lead to a student being stigmatized socially are a high treatment priority. To illustrate, a lisp and [w] for [r] are often early treatment sounds because they may provoke teasing. Impact of an error on intelligibility also influences sound selection. Errors that negatively affect intelligibility are good candidates for treatment. These include deletions, changes in place of production, and substitutions in the beginning of words.

Treatment

Three Questions

Before selecting treatment resources, at least three questions must be resolved:

- How many sounds should be treated?
- What constitutes a correct production of a treatment sound?
- Should a student be stimulable for a treatment sound?

How Many Sounds to Treat?

The assessment typically yields one or more possible treatment sounds. This raises the following questions:

- If a student's speech contains more than one possibility, which sound to select?
- Should one sound be worked on to completion and then another?
- Should two be worked on simultaneously, changing from one to another in the same treatment session or in alternate sessions?
- Does working on two or more treatment sounds confuse a student?

The author's view is that answers to these questions have more to do with human variables than linguistic factors. Some students—especially older ones—

can work on a sound from beginning to completion, while others benefit from alternating between sounds, sometimes within a single treatment session, sometimes in alternate sessions. A useful dynamic assessment is to initially select several treatment sounds, alternating between them either in a single session or in alternate sessions, and then re-evaluate the choice after several treatment sessions.

What Constitutes a Correct Production of a Treatment Sound?

Whenever possible, treatment should avoid practicing a speech error—something the student probably already has lots of practice doing! Ideally, a sound should be entirely correct during practice. An analogy might be: suppose a coach wanted to teach a student a new tennis stroke. Ideally, the coach wants to establish the stroke perfectly and then engage in perfect practice. However, in both speech-language pathology and tennis, sometimes something less than ideal is accepted, and both a clinician and a coach may need to practice a skill that is better than before, but still not perfect. For this reason, a "3," "2," "1" rather than a "correct/incorrect" system often proves useful (Highnam, 2004). A student's old speech pattern is a "3," and the goal is to establish it as a "1" (perfect). However, in many instances a "3" does not automatically become "1," and, instead, the student produces something like a "2"— a more correct version of the old pattern, but one still not perfect. Speech treatment often contains many more "2"s than "1"s. While practicing a less than perfect sound the student learns to make it a "1" through self-reflection activities and prompts.

Should a Student Be Stimulable for a Treatment Sound?

An important, much debated question is will a student self-correct stimulable sounds without treatment (Dietrich, 1983; Powell, 1991; Powell, Elbert, & Dinnsen, 1991; Shine, 1989)? Research suggests extensive individual variation, with some students self-correcting and others not. Some clinicians choose to work with only stimulable sounds and others select only to treat nonstimuable ones. Many other clinicians fall in the middle, working first on a stimulable sound to build a student's confidence before tackling more difficult nonstimulable sounds.

In general, the author prefers to teach stimulable sounds. A useful "trick of the trade," especially with a younger or less motivated student, is to first treat a stimuable sound to help build confidence before attempting the more challenging nonstimulable sounds. However, selecting a stimulable sound often is not an option for an older school-aged student (typically, preteens and teenagers) or an adult nonnative speaker. In this situation, a nonstimulable sound is selected for treatment.

A challenging situation can arise if a preteen or teenager with a nonstimulable sound is an unwilling participant in therapy, "forced" to receive treatment by parents or teachers. In this situation, after an initial period of therapy a student may be placed on a semester by semester contract in which continued treatment is dependent on a student's effort and success. The purpose of the contract is to avoid a difficult situation in which an unmotivated student continues in therapy semester after semester, bored, demoralized, and unsuccessful. Better a therapeutic break than a broken spirit!

> ### *Stimulability and Religion*
>
> In the absence of research clearly supporting one position or the other, the discussion of stimulability at times almost seems religious, some fervently asserting this and others just as fervently asserting that. An alternative to accepting one or the other position is to be your own researcher, experimenting with different perspectives. Perhaps you will find that you have more success with nonstimulable sounds than reported by some, or perhaps you will have less. Or perhaps you will discover which students on your caseload seem to require a treatment sound that is stimulable and which do not. No matter what you discover, experimenting with different approaches may yield important insights about what works best for you and the students you serve.

Once a sound or sounds have been selected for treatment, the following resources are used:

- Metaphors
- Touch cues
- Demonstrations
- Phonetic placement and shaping techniques
- Key environments
- Word lists
- Awareness and speech exercises
- Language activities

Metaphors, Touch Cues, and Demonstrations

Metaphors, touch cues, and demonstrations all provide useful ways to refer to treatment sounds, and especially during early treatment phases may help focus a student on the task at hand. As treatment progresses, they serve as reminders and prompts.

Metaphors

Metaphors provide useful analogies for a treatment sound. Typically, a clinician presents several possible metaphors, allowing a student to select between them. With a younger student, the metaphors make analogy with something familiar—perhaps an engine starting, a hissing snake, or a leaky tire. With an older student the metaphors often refer to an aspect of the treatment sound—that is, an interdental may be the tongue-out sound, [s] with a lowered tongue tip may be the tongue-down sound, or [l] may be the pointy sound. For a student who is a teenager or an adult, many times a treatment sound is called by its technical name. To illustrate, with an adult student a clinician may decide to call [s] "a fricative sound" or "a fricative made at the alveolar ridge."

Often, a metaphor proves more successful when a student helps select it. Typically, a clinician presents several options and asks the student to select one. Allowing a student to help select a metaphor entails the clinician giving up a measure of control—after all, a student is not obliged to select the metaphor that the clinician thinks best captures the nature of the speech problem. A clinician weighs selection of the most appropriate metaphor against a student's need for involvement. In the author's experience, most often the issue does not arise and selection of a metaphor presents few problems. If a question of appropriateness versus student involvement arose, most clinicians give up the best, most appropriate metaphor in favor of student involvement.

Touch Cues

Touch cues are finger positions that represent a treatment sound, allowing a clinician to refer to a treatment sound using modalities other than speech. Touch cues grossly mimic speech movements. An older student understands that, for example, the touch cue for velar consonants is made parallel to the back of the mouth, representing where the tongue is raised. A younger student may benefit from a touch cue without realizing its mimicking quality. For such a student, a touch cue is a visual and tactile reminder, a way to say, "Remember: this is the sound we are working on."

Demonstrations

Demonstrations show a student how a treatment sound is produced. By drawing attention to such aspects of speech as tongue position and airflow a student may better understand how to pronounce a treatment sound. Older students often find demonstrations intellectually engaging and interesting. Others, especially those under 7 years, may find demonstrations more confusing than helpful. Demonstrations find their most use early in treatment. Later in treatment, an occasional demonstration may serve as a reminder about how a treatment sound is produced.

Phonetic Placement and Shaping Techniques

Phonetic placement techniques show a student how to place the articulators to pronounce a sound, and shaping techniques show a student how to convert one sound into another. These techniques are used when a nonstimulable sound is selected for treatment. Students seven years or older typically possess sufficient attention and language skills to benefit from these techniques. With a younger student success with these techniques is more hit-or-miss. The techniques are typically inappropriate (and ineffective) with a child under 4 years.

Though every clinician has favorite phonetic placement and shaping technique, no single technique works for every student. In general, a clinician selects one that makes intuitive sense and then engages in trial-and-error dynamic assessment. Often, from a few to 5 to 10 minutes is sufficient to determine if a particular technique will prove successful. In general, when selecting a technique, most clinicians prefer those that are simpler and have shorter instructions. Longer techniques are turned to when the shorter, simpler ones do not yield results.

The phonetic placement and shaping techniques listed in this book are "bare bones recipes" to expand and modify as a clinician desires. Often, the actual phonetic placement or shaping technique used with a student contains the following elements:

1. An initial self-demonstration by the clinician.
2. The student practices the steps in the technique. Use of a touch cue and metaphors focus the student and help remind him or her about how the sound is pronounced.
3. The student attempts to make the sound.
4. The clinician gives feedback about the success of the attempt.

The following illustrates one possible way to fully expand a bare bones phonetic placement technique:

Phonetic Placement Technique for [θ]

Objects: Feather or small piece of paper

Instructions:

1. First demonstrate the method on yourself.
2. To begin, place your tongue between your upper and lower front teeth.
3. Place a feather or small piece of paper in front of your mouth, about a half-inch to an inch from your tongue.
4. Blow air over your tongue to move the feather or paper.

5. Explain, "That's how you make the leaking tire sound. Now it's your turn."
6. Instruct the student to stick out his or her tongue just as you did.
7. When the tongue is out, place the feather or paper before the mouth.
8. Explain, "Now blow to make it move."
9. If the sound is made correctly, say, "That's right. You did it. You made [θ]— the leaky tire sound." If the sound is made incorrectly, say something like, "Good try. Let's try again."

Key Environments

Key environments describe phonetic environments in which a student is likely to pronounce a sound correctly. In addition to being used during the evaluation to determine if a student has the capacity to make a sound, key environments find good use after a treatment sound (or sounds) is selected, providing a possible succession of environments in which to treat a sound. The following illustrates how key environments might be used to establish [s], [l], and [r] in the beginning of words, end of words, between vowels, and in consonant clusters.

Beginning of Word

Establish [s], [l], and [r] before a high front vowel. Once established, expand the number of different vowels that follow. For a student that is strongly affected by the adjacent vowel, back high vowels are likely to be more challenging than front ones.

End of Word

[s] is more likely to be established here than [l] and [r]. Establish after a high front vowel. Next, to make word-initial sounds, have the word-final sounds be followed by a word beginning with a vowel, such as "bus and." This encourages the sound to "migrate" to start the following word, resulting in, for example, "bu sand."

Between Vowels

[l] and [r] are more likely to be established here than [s], though some students find [s] easier to make here, too. For all three consonants, establish between two high front vowels, as in *ili*. Once established, add different adjacent vowels. To expand to word-initial position, have the student drop the first vowel, resulting in, for example, [li]. To expand to word-final position, follow the same procedure, resulting in, for example, [il].

Consonant Clusters

For [s], establish after [t] as in "pizza" or the nonsense word [tsi]. To expand the environments in which [s] occurs, have [ts] be followed by different vowels. To help expand [s] to syllable-initial position, encourage the student to drop the [t]. For [l] and [r], establish after a consonant with a different place of production than [l] and [r] (most often, select [p] or [b]) followed by a high front vowel. Next, to help expand [l] and [r] ask the student to drop the initial consonant in the consonant cluster.

Word Lists

Word lists are used to generate stimuli to help establish a sound in a student's speech, and then to practice it. Words, rather than nonsense syllables, are the vehicle for teaching a treatment sound for two reasons:

1. Words, carefully selected, offer relatively simple phonetic contexts in which to teach a sound, and
2. Words, being a student's everyday means of communication, are used both in and outside of treatment, making them a critical bridge to generalization.

Word lists in this book are divided by phonetic environment; in the accompanying DVD lists of minimal pairs, deletions, and themes also are included. Word lists are therapeutic building blocks for many different exercises and activities. The value of using isolated words diminishes as treatment proceeds and the clinician shifts to more naturalistic activities.

Awareness and Speech Exercises

Awareness exercises focus a student's attention on the treatment sound. They are used frequently early in therapy to orient a student, and later in therapy may be used primarily as prompts and reminders.

Speech exercises help a student to gain experience with a treatment sound, providing practice in pronouncing, self-monitoring, and self-correcting speech. The most frequently used exercises are imitation, minimal pairs, deletions, multiple productions, old way/new way, and similar sounds. Speech exercises are used most often in language activities and, less frequently, as a list of words. Many times a mix of exercises is used. For example, a student may be asked to delete the treatment sound and then say the word with the treatment sound three times.

> ### *Discrimination Versus Awareness*
>
> The difference between discrimination exercises and awareness exercises lies in conception, not actually practice. If a reader prefers, awareness exercises described in this book may be used as and called discrimination exercises. However, within the author's perspective the conceptual distinction between discrimination and awareness is important. The term *discrimination* implies a student's difficulty lies in the auditory system's inability to distinguish between sounds; however, research strongly suggests that the auditory system, in common with other sensory systems, matures early, and has adultlike capacities near the end of a child's first year (Pascallis, de Haan, & Nelson; 2002). The term *awareness* implies the therapeutic challenge is to focus a student's attention on the difference between an intended pronunciation and what actually comes out of the mouth. A student with a speech problem, like most other persons, is not likely to closely monitor his or her speech even when what comes out the mouth differs considerably from the speech of the community. An awareness exercise is a little verbal tap on the shoulder, saying "Remember what sound you are working on. Focus on what you are doing."

Language Activities

Language activities use school books and other outside materials, including stories a student is reading, favorite stories from home, and articles from newspapers and magazines. These materials, because they are familiar and widely used, are easy to adapt by families, aides, and teachers. Many times their use also has the practical advantage of improving a student's academic skills. Though the purpose of therapy is speech, much is gained if in the process of learning speech a student also does better on classroom assignments or gives a better oral report.

Summary

The discussion in this chapter illustrates *one way* care might be conceptualized and carried out. Within this perspective, treatment for late-acquired sounds is conceptualized as helping a student learn new ways of speaking and to unlearn old ones. This requires a treatment approach focusing on both the articulation and phonologic aspects of speech. Within this view, a treatment program focused solely on articulation is like a building a train that doesn't actually go anywhere, while a treatment program focused solely on phonology is like a destination without a vehicle to get there. Treatment of late-acquired sounds requires careful attention to building a good train to reach a worthwhile travel destination. An additional characteristic of this framework is that human variables such as motivation, intelligence, family support, attention, and desire to learn are recognized as being at least equally important for clinical success as linguistic ones. Lastly, the framework emphasizes the importance of using functional activities that contribute to the advancement of a student's education and social development.

References

Bleile, K. (2004). *A manual of articulation and phonological disorders* (2nd ed.). Clifton Park, NY: Delmar Thomson.

Diedrich, W. (1983). Stimulability and articulation disorders. In J. Locke (Ed.), *Seminars in Speech and Language, 4.*

Highnam, D. (2004). Personal communication.

Pascallis, O., de Haan, M., & Nelson, C. (2002). Is face processing species-specific during the first year of life? *Science, 296*, 1321-1323.

Powell, T. (1991). Planning for phonological generalization: An approach to treatment target selection. *American Journal of Speech Language Pathology, 1*, 21-27.

Powell, T., Elbert, M., & Dinnsen, D. (1991). Stimulability as a factor in the phonological generalization of misarticulating preschool children. *Journal of Speech and Hearing Research, 34*, 1318-1328.

Shine, R. (1989). Articulatory production training: A sensory-motor approach. In N. Creaghead, P. Newman, & W. Secord (Eds.), *Assessment and remediation of articulatory and phonological disorders* (pp. 355-359). Columbus, OH: Charles E. Merrill.

Chapter 12

Motor Learning Guided Therapy

Carlin Hageman

Introduction

Teaching a young child to produce speech to match the culturally accepted norm is no easy feat. True, some children seem to be natural pleasers who will do anything that you suggest. Others tend to go along with you when there seems to be a good reason to do it. Finally, there are children who actively resist practicing new ways of talking, perhaps because they cannot see the point or because they just do not place practicing speech at a higher priority than fooling around. This chapter will not provide you with a magic bullet to reach all of those children, but it may provide you with the tools to modify your therapy so that the child learns the most he or she can in the few minutes you have for practice. That is important because we are under great pressure to produce better results, in a shorter time, using fewer resources. Therefore, the goal of this chapter is to help you plan therapy that has the potential to address those demands.

Many of us have attempted to learn a new motor skill or one that was difficult. Some of us have tried to teach or coach young learners to play a musical instrument or master an athletic skill. As speech-language pathologists, we are concerned about teaching articulatory skills (motor skills) to young children who have failed to learn how to articulate the sounds of the language. This chapter addresses the motor learning components of articulation while fully realizing that articulation is just one component of the complicated system of linguistic and motor competences.

Much of what is known about motor learning arises from disciplines other than speech pathology, and little literature exists that examines the principles of motor learning in speech. In my opinion, it is crucial that speech-language pathologists explore new ways of thinking about therapy to make our therapy more efficient and more likely to engender carry-over to real world communication. Thus, I have chosen to utilize the principles of motor learning—Motor Learning Guided (MLG)—to structure practice, knowing full well that all of the principles are not yet delineated in their relative efficiencies and inefficiencies with respect to articulation.

> ### *Thinking About It*
>
> Have we ever delineated all of the procedures and processes that we currently use (e.g., immediate or constant feedback)? Have we considered if behavior modification is the correct model for practice of a motor skill? Do our traditional methods work? Of course they do for many learners, but are they suitable for everyone and the most efficient and cost effective?

Motor Skill

Motor Control

Clearly, all of us have learned motor skills in a variety of domains to greater and lesser degrees. Some of us have amazing aptitudes for certain motor skills; the athlete or musician who seems to be able to accomplish any complex feat of athletic skill or perform the most complex musical pieces. On the other hand, most of us are able to accomplish the most amazing athletic feat of all—we talk. For example, Netsell (1991) noted that speech required a minimum of 140,000 neuromuscular events per second (14 phonemes per second × 100 muscles × 100 motor units per muscle). It is a remarkable achievement that most of us attain. Why do some children find talking so difficult and some find it almost impossible to acquire. For example, the causes are relatively apparent in the children with motor speech disorders and hearing loss. In others, the underlying causes are not obvious. For the present discussion, we are going to consider that the process of motor learning is disrupted, and discuss the variables that we, as speech-language pathologists, can control in the context of practice for learning to speak.

> ### *Thinking About It*
> What could disrupt motor learning of articulation? What are the necessary capabilities for learning the skill of speaking?

Although it is not certain that learning to talk is affected by the same principles that have been shown to be effective for motor learning in other domains, it is certain that speech is a highly complex motor skill and that we can speak "automatically" with little effort or attention directed to the motor control aspects of speaking. Since the effort is low to control the motor aspect of speech for most of us, we can attend to the social context, linguistic structure, and communicative intent. Controlling complex motor activities with low effort suggests that speech may be controlled by motor programs that are automatic mechanisms of motor control. Is there evidence for programmatic control of speech? One example was provided by Robin et al. (2008) who demonstrated that normal speakers, speakers with apraxia of speech or dysarthria, differ in their ability to track a moving target with their jaw, lips, and voice. Essentially, apraxic speakers could not track a predictable target as well as normal or dysarthric speakers. On the other hand, the apraxic speakers could track an unpredictable signal as well as the normal or dysarthric speakers because all three groups used closed-loop control (nonprogrammatic) for unpredictable targets. The findings were interpreted as evidence for motor programming in the control of speech. Backlin et al. (2008) and Gaughan, Howard, and Hageman (2009), using a speech inhibition task, found evidence of programmatic or automatic control of speech in adults and children.

Closed Loop and Open Loop

Schmidt and Wrisberg (2004) described two methods of motor control—closed-loop and open-loop control. Closed loop is characterized by slow movements because the movements are constantly modified by sensory feedback about the movement and the environment. Closed-loop control is slow and effort is intensive; consequently, too slow to control the fast movements of speech. In contrast, during open-loop control, the performer recalls a set of instructions (or programs) for controlling muscle movements that, once initiated, are completed without modification. Open-loop control systems are fast because the movements (instructions) are completed without modification. The disadvantage of open-loop control is that when the environment changes, the performer is unable to change the movement once it has been initiated or if the wrong movement is planned, it is likely to be executed before the performer can stop it. Since the open-loop control system demands low effort or attention, the performer can pay attention to the environmental demand (e.g., listeners) and plan subsequent movements.

Because nearly all movements occur within unique contexts, do skilled performers remember all possible movements or programs? Schmidt and Wrisberg (2004) pointed out that memory limitation preclude that possibility and developed schema theory to complement the notion of general motor programs. Although this is not a suitable venue for a lengthy discussion of their model, a basic understanding is necessary in order to understand the principles of motor learning. The reader is referred to Maas et al. (2008) for a detailed review of schema theory and to Schmidt and Wrisberg (2004) for complete explanation.

Schema Theory

Underlying schema theory is an assumption that there are units of motor activity (motor programs) and that these motor programs (MP) are stored and retrieved from memory and adapted to the specific requirements of the moment (Schmidt, 1988; Schmidt & Wrisberg, 2004). These MPs have invariant and variant features. The invariant features include the temporal relationships between components (timing) and order of events. The variant features consist of elements of a movement that can vary (e.g., absolute speed, loudness). The size of the unit in speech has not been specified for certain, but Stetson (1951) hypothesized that it was the syllable. Carr (2004) demonstrated that invariant feature control across at least three syllables was present in young children as early as 5 years (i.e., the children maintained relative timing and order across rates of speech). Although the syllable may be a core feature of speech, it would seem that speech motor programs can be longer than one syllable. Backlin et al. (2008) and Gaughan, Howard, and Hageman (2009) found that program length was at least two to three syllables in length in adults using a refractory time test. Because speech consists of nearly an infinite variety of phoneme and syllable combinations and given the infinite array of initial conditions, goals, and motor modalities, it is not possible to remember all programs. Schmidt (1988) proposed that the programs are generalized and then organized for the specific act needed.

Once the intent to speak has arisen, schema theory suggests that certain processes must occur (Figure 12–1). The motor control system of the performer must be aware of initial conditions, both internal and external (e.g., the structures involved in the movement and the characteristics of the environment relevant to the goal). For example, in golf, the player is knowledgeable (though not necessarily cognitively aware) of the muscular system status, joint positions (internal), and target place (external), and the recall schema uses this information to recall a GMP and predicts the outcome of the movement. Once the movement is generated, the information is stored in the recognition schema where the outcome of the movements, the prediction of the movements, and the consequences (both internal and external) are compared to the actual outcomes (internal and external). When there is a mismatch between the predicted external (desired) outcomes, the learner can tweak the GMP to attempt to make the next movement more accurate or examine the intended internal sensations

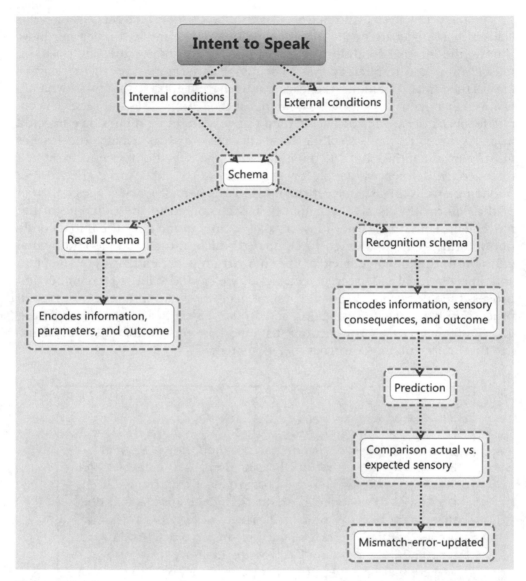

Figure 12-1. Processes hypothesized to occur when intent to speak is formed.

to ensure that the intended movement was actually completed. In a sense, the learner uses the errors to create a better GMP for the next attempt, either for the specification of the invariant features of the plan (stay the same across many different iterations of the movement) or the variant features of the plan (vary with specifics of the target [e.g., greater force]). From this writer's perspective, we can hypothesize influences that may create problems for the learner.

First, if the learner does not have an idea of the correct target, practice attempts are not modifiable. For example, a deaf child or a child with auditory processing problems may not have a clear notion of speech targets. Second, the learner must be aware of the initial conditions. For example, the learner must "know" the internal conditions (e.g., the position of the tongue, jaw position, muscle tone, and respiratory system status). Furthermore, even if the learner knows the initial conditions, the learner must have feedback about the dynamic changes that occur during the movements. If the learner does not receive accurate feedback or no feedback at all, then the next attempt will not be corrected in any systematic way—resulting in nearly random trials. Finally, the learner must be aware of the external conditions, meaning, whether the movement had intended consequences on or for the target (e.g., did I make the correct phoneme or did the listener get the message). Schema theory suggests that all of this information is held in memory and compared to the outcome of the movement. Thus, the learner must be able to hold in memory the initial condition information long enough to compare (which also takes time and mental effort) it to the outcome. Hence, the comparison is dependent upon accurate and timely internal and external feedback as well as the ability to remember and process the information. Factors that have been shown to interfere with mental processing may include distraction and arousal levels that are too high or too low (Kahneman, 1973). The sections that follow are this author's attempts to utilize this information to construct therapy practice.

> ### *Thinking About It*
>
> Do we have diagnostic tests for these variables. Hearing—certainly is available for hearing across the frequency spectrum but maybe not for dynamic hearing. Internal conditions—no, for ability to know tactically, kinesthetically, and so forth, the conditions of the speech production mechanism. What does that mean? Perhaps for some learners, we are making serious errors that they know "articulatory movements." And no, for testing the ability to hold in working memory the motor plan and compare it to results. What about attention? Do we measure the learner's ability to attend to information about a movement long enough to make adjustments to the plan and commit the adjustments to memory.

Principles of Motor Learning

Learning Versus Acquisition

Before we delve into the specifics of motor learning applied to speech practice, we need to make the distinction between acquisition performance and learning.

Acquisition performance refers to the momentary strength of a pattern (skill) during practice; whereas, learning refers to what the learner remembers at a point remote from the practice. This can be measured as retention, generalization, and spread. The important point for this discussion is that during acquisition (practice), both the learner and the therapist will do things to improve performance during practice that will be detrimental to retention or generalization (e.g., constant feedback with description and cuing). More will be said about this in the feedback section. Learning can also be inhibited during practice by constant evaluation, which may affect arousal levels. Many of us have seen the anxious child looking over our shoulder trying to catch a glimpse of the scores (Hageman, Mueller, Burda, & Bleile, 2004; Maas et al., 2008; Schmidt & Wrisberg, 2004).

Thinking About It

What is the purpose of saying "good job" after each trial? What are the consequences of praise after each trial? When is the learner allowed to make the internal comparisons about the adequacy of the movement? How much time is necessary to make that comparison? What capabilities does the learner need to have to make those comparisons and use them? How or when does clinician behavior interfere with learning?

Prepractice

Before practice begins, the learner should be prepared for practice (Schmidt & Lee, 2005). Maas et al. (2008) suggested three goals of prepractice including: (a) motivation to learn, (b) adequate understanding of the task including a basic knowledge of correct, and (c) stimulability for acceptable responses to avoid frustration. Although I think these are worthy goals, in my experience, it is important not to expect prepractice attempts to be accurate before practice begins. For me, it is more important that the learner is able to vary the productions. As a clinician, one must broaden acceptable responses to include the ability to systematically vary movements even when they are incorrect with respect to the "correct" response.

As part of the prepractice time, it is important to gather information about the invariant and variant features of the learner's speech. The invariant features include the rhythm or prosody of the utterances including the relative durations of segments and the order of the movements. Several researchers, including Schmidt and Wrisberg (2004) and Schmidt and Lee (2005) have observed that practice addressing the invariant features should precede the practice with the variant features (i.e., articulation of individual sounds).

> ### *Thinking About It*
>
> To learn to throw a baseball or softball, it is necessary to learn the order of movements before worrying about accuracy of the throw (e.g., correct starting point, opposite leg motion, rotation of the hips, then rotation of shoulders, then the arm forward motion, and then the wrist snap). What about speech? What are the correct starting positions? What is the first movement, the second, and so on. How much relative time should those movements consume? Do we test or observe these events?

Selecting goals is another important aspect of pre-practice. In my approach to motor learning guided practice, I try to keep it simple and designate the learner as either an early learner or an advanced learner. The point is that goals for early learners should be more performance oriented (e.g., better lip position) and advanced learners should be more results oriented (e.g., correct phoneme). Above all, the goals should be within reach of the learner.

Understanding the task is an element of prepractice that has several dimensions. For an adult with a motor speech disorder, Maas et al. (2008) recommends that the learner be provided with a reference of correctness and explanations of why it is correct or not. From my perspective, explanations using details about the error, the nature of the error, or mechanism of the error add too much cognitive load to the learning process. Most of us have probably experienced the zealous coach or instructor who overwhelmed us with detail until we were paralyzed by analysis. One common trick to play on a fellow golfer is to ask: "Do you always hold your fingers that way?" Maas et al. (2008) cautioned us to avoid complex, lengthy explanations and to use instructions that match the comprehension abilities of the learner. Most of us probably could recall providing instructions and feedback that were more complex than the task the learner was practicing.

Practice

Mass et al. (2008) provided an outstanding breakdown of the different ways that practice can be addressed and it is beyond the scope of this chapter to go into detail about each one. Figure 12–2 shows many elements that may influence motor learning. In general, the more practice the better, but you must take into account fatigue, which detracts from the benefit of practice. In addition, large amounts of constant practice are contraindicated. Consequently, practice distribution is an important consideration, especially in early learners for whom fatigue or motivation may be a problem.

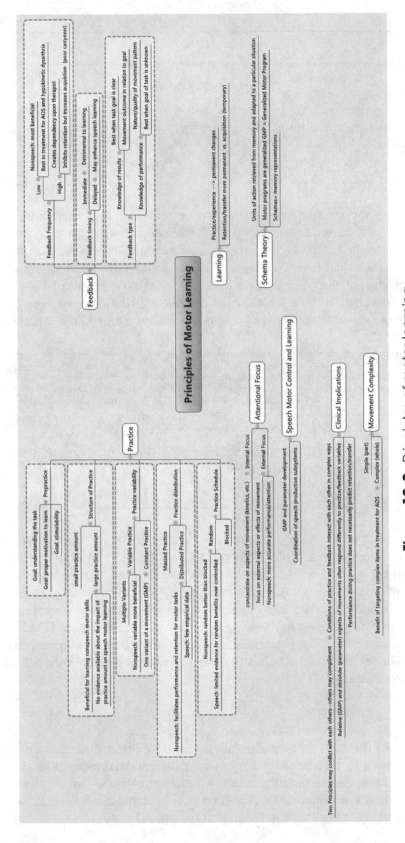

Figure 12-2. Principles of motor learning.

> ### *Thinking About It*
>
> Why does fatigue affect practice? Does it affect attention through low arousal, which means that focused attention is difficult? Does it mean the learner loses interest and does not "tweak" the motor plan after a trial using mental effort?

Variable practice has been shown to be superior for enhancing learning during practice. In a sense, the less predictable the practice items are, the more challenging the task. Guadagnoli and Lee reported increased difficulty during practice enhances learning (Guadagnoli & Lee, 2004). Other research has shown that forcing the learner to generate a plan for each practice attempt has positive effects on learning. In fact, Schmidt and Wrisberg (2004) have reported that even imaging (visualizing) the movement has positive effects on learning.

> ### *Thinking About It*
>
> We defined motor learning as what the learner remembers how to do at a time remote from the practice. If you score acquisition behavior (i.e., during practice), the tendency is to simplify practice, provide more feedback and cuing to achieve higher acquisition scores, but that comes at the price of poorer retention.

Using random practice can be more beneficial for learning than blocked practice. In our experience, blocked practice may be more effective for the early learners whereas random practice is more effective for the advanced learner. However, when we use blocked practice, we do not allow rapid repetitions of the production. We impose delays of up to 5 seconds between reiterations of the practice item. During the pause, we do not allow the learner to talk, play games, or fidget because we have hypothesized that one variable underlying the poor learning of speech is a lack of attention devoted to the recognition schema and modification of the GMP.

Focus

Where should the learner focus his/her attention during practice? The learner has two options in that he/she can focus on the internal aspects of the movement (e.g., kinesthetic, kinematic, and somatosensory as in the feel of the tongue during the production of the /r/) or the external aspects (e.g., how does the /r/ sound or how does the listener respond). The evidence is very strong that an external focus produces a strong advantage for learning in the non-speech motor domain. The movements tend to be more accurate and less variable but even so there may be some interaction between the level of performance (new or more experienced learner) and the task (Wulf, Shea, & McNevin, 2003).

> ### *Thinking About It*
>
> This issue may lie at the heart of some children trying to learn to speak. When clinicians suggest that attention be directed to the feel of the act, they assume that the mechanisms of perception are normal. Our current state of the art does not allow us to test those senses. Because the movements of the pharynx, velum, and tongue essentially are invisible to the learner, poor sensory ability to detect, identify, and remember sensations of speech may make internal focus of feedback and instruction frustrating. On the other hand, some ability to know what the structures are doing is necessary or the next try is essentially random.

External focus is thought to enhance learning because the learner is not encouraged to constrain the motor system through conscious control and the more automatic motor response is encouraged. One could also think of this as a conflict of open- versus closed-loop control. Paying attention to internal characteristics is effort-intensive and slow, thus encouraging the use of a closed-loop control system, which is neurophysiologically different from open-loop control. Consequently, one would not expect a great deal of learning or generalization to automatic performance.

However, since external versus internal control of speech movements has not been investigated up to this point, we have to make some assumptions. First, we know that speech movements are highly complex and fast. Second, we know that speakers proceed with talking with little effort allocated to the internal aspects of speech. Consequently, at present, I am willing to assume that speech has more in common with rapid, complex nonspeech movements than not. I am going to suggest that we stress external focus to our clients. Thus, what does the speech sound like and what is the effect on the environment? Turning our clients into "mini" speech-language pathologists with the complicated explanations is counterproductive because it directs their attention to internal factors, which require too much effort to utilize during speech production. This advice is not pervasive because a learner who did not know how to start producing a sound may need some advice about the starting position and first movement articulatory movement.

Feedback

From my perspective, traditional articulation therapy mixes up feedback with
reinforcement. Operant reinforcement strategies are utilized to increase or
decrease behaviors by providing immediate reinforcement or punishment.
Operant techniques clearly have a role in therapy, especially behavioral manage-
ment, but they should not be confused with feedback.

Feedback is information about the performance or the outcome of the performance. Two sources of feedback are possible (see Figure 12–2). Internal feedback is what the performer can discern from his/her own senses about the
results of the movement and about the movement itself. External feedback is
information supplied to the performer by a coach or therapist. Schmidt and
Wrisbert (2004) were emphatic that external feedback that duplicates that
which the performer can perceive, has a neutral effect at best and more commonly is detrimental to learning. Consider how irritating it would be for a coach
to keep telling you that you made the basket when you can see that you did (literature is clear that too high arousal levels interfere with learning). In addition,
Schmidt and Wrisberg (2004) reported that excessive feedback contributes to
dependency on the coach or therapist for correct performance rather than internal direction or evaluation.

> is not the same as giving feedback. Using cognitive "questioning," like how did that feel, and so forth, is counterproductive because it misdirects attention and effort involved in evaluating performance and is a difficult cognitive task (e.g., can you put into words how it feels to elevate your velum during speech?)

On the other hand, when internal feedback mechanisms are absent or deficient, then the coach or therapist must provide the information. Schmidt and Wrisberg (2004) described two types of external feedback: knowledge of results (KR) and knowledge of performance (KP). KR is information about the result of the movement in the world (e.g., that sound was correct). KP is information about the performance of movement (e.g., your lips were too rounded). My experience with traditional practice structure has led me to believe that KP and KR are used much too frequently and that little consideration is given to whether the learner can discern the information without feedback. So, where does that leave the clinician?

The principles of motor learning have not yet been investigated to the point where specific rules and guidelines can be proposed for the use of feedback for speech practice. Following Schmidt and Wrisberg (2004), with respect to feedback, less is more and delayed is better. In other words, the clinician should strive to use only the feedback that the learner needs and make the learner wait for it. The clinician must use his/her best clinical judgment to determine the needs of the learner.

> ### *Thinking About It*
>
> Why make the learner wait for it? From my perspective, I am hypothesizing that with practice the learner may begin to be able to use internal feedback. Forcing him or her to wait for KR or KP may provide an opportunity to use that internal feedback and give the learner time to compare the actual movement/result with what was intended. Of course, with this model you run the risk of duplication of what the learner can do. Limiting the frequency of feedback may address that issue.

For example, it is obvious that the deaf child needs KR certainly; however, it is not so obvious that the deaf child needs KP. The deaf child would need KP providing that he/she could not perceive the movements that led to the KR received. Furthermore, even KR would not be needed provided the child could discern the reaction of the environment to the attempted production. In other words, when the child can determine if the production resulted in the desired effect in the real world, then he/she would not need to be told. Of course, during practice, it might take considerable ingenuity by the clinician to create communication interactions that lead to independent judgments by the learner rather than just direct feedback from the clinician. At this point, the clinician should use every tool available to determine what the learner can perceive.

Since few, if any, tools are available to the clinician to measure a child's ability to perceive the position and movement of the articulators, we need to go back to the model of the schema whereby the learner modifies behavior by comparing what he/she intended to do with what actually occurred and then evaluating the effect on the environment. If the learner, in our case, the child is unable to acquire and remember internal and accurate feedback about the results and the movement, then the comparison cannot be made in order to adjust the next trial. External feedback is then required.

How frequent should the feedback be? A few investigations have examined the frequency of feedback in speech (e.g., Kim, LaPointe, & Stierwalt, 2012; Steinhauer & Preston Grayhack, 2000; Wambaugh, Kalinyak-Flizzar, West, & Doyle, 1998). Consistently, they have demonstrated that feedback between 20% and 60% is more effective for retention than 100% percent feedback. However, for the tasks they examined, they did not control for learner experience. In other words, in keeping with Schmidt and Wrisberg's (2004) notions, if the learners were just beginning, 100% feedback might be appropriate for a few trials.

How precise should the feedback be? Schmidt and Wrisberg (2004) described several types of feedback; among them are summary feedback, average feedback, and bandwidth feedback. Their guiding principle was that feedback should be as vague as possible so that the learner is forced to figure it out. An example of bandwidth feedback might be that the production of /l/ fell between an /r/ and /w/ sounds. Average feedback is also quite vague. The therapist might describe a set of five practice trials, as on the whole, those were pretty good. In summary mode, the therapist might report that the first two were accurate, the third and fourth were inaccurate, and the fifth one was inaccurate. The size of the set about which to give feedback is dependent on the learner's experience. However, Hageman et al. (2004) described a therapy trial in which the feedback was provided to an apraxic child about vowels and consonants; however, the child was not told which she was receiving, that is, vowel or consonant feedback. The child was able to figure it out and had remarkable improvement in her speech accuracy.

Another important variable to control during practice is the post-KR delay interval (Hall, Jordan, & Robin, 1993). Hageman et al. (2004) expanded on the post-KR delay interval notion to include postproduction delay interval. The purpose of these delays was to provide time for the learner to process the internal feedback (postproduction) and then to process the external feedback (post-KR or KP). The assumption being made was that the learner needed that time to compare the intended movement, with the actual movement, and then with the consequences of the movement in the environment (internal and external feedback).

In some investigations we have used as much as 5 seconds of delay and as little as 1 second. The entire range has shown to produce learning; however, we do not know the optimum time. In fact, it may not be the delay that is critical but rather the enforced "quiet time" that allows for attention to be allocated to the comparison task, followed by GMP tweaking. It is not necessarily externally directed attention but rather a period of time in which the neurological processes of recalling a program, remembering the program, and comparing the program with the results of the movement can occur. For example, in one study, the learner was consistently vocally rehearsing (groping) an incorrect production during the postproduction interval, which we interpreted to show that he was not making the necessary comparisons but was engaging in rapid trial and error experimentation. When we enforced the quiet delay postproduction, he began to show improvement (Hageman, 2005, clinical observation).

Measurement

Every day as I interact in my clinic, I hear supervisors and students interacting about "taking data." Since I was in graduate school, "taking data" has meant judging each performance as it is made and entering the "score" on a variety of forms. However, Schmidt and Wrisberg (2004) and others have described in depth the problems with this approach to measuring learning. These problems are serious and interfere with learning and our interpretation of what the learner actually knows.

We must make a distinction between the momentary strength of a behavior (acquisition) versus the permanent memory (retention) of a behavior. This distinction is important because both the clinician and the learner will do things that improve acquisition scores but reduce retention. We have worried about this issue for years, calling it carryover. There are at least three aspects of permanent learning that we should consider. Retention is measured by performance on the practiced tasks at some time remote from the practice (e.g., at the next session). Generalization is measured by performance on tasks that are closely related to the practiced task (e.g., unpracticed words with the targeted sounds). Social validation is determined by measuring the use of the learning targets in normal day-to-day activities. The key element is that none of these measures is completed during practice.

Why is measurement remote in time necessary? First, measurement during practice typically increases arousal and anxiety. Increased arousal levels are detrimental to learning particularly in new or sensitive learners. (Importantly,

I think it also detracts from the clinician's ability to manage the therapeutic milieu as it is a divided attention task.) Second, measurement during practice encourages clinicians to use strategies that increase practice scores (e.g., blocked practice, constant feedback, etc.) but negatively impact retention. Third, learners will attempt to use as little variability as possible to maintain accuracy, which does increase acquisition scores but decreases retention score.

Consequently, I recommend that retention testing be completed periodically. How often is that? Well, it depends. One should consider the learning level of the client. More experienced learners could be measured less frequently whereas new learners could be measured once each session. For generalization and social validation, perhaps even longer time intervals would be more appropriate. The intervals are unique to individuals and depend on rate of learning and the demands of third-party interests.

Movement Complexity

Because we already have established that speech is a remarkably complex and rapid set of movements, what is there about speech complexity that can be managed to promote learning? Let's examine rate. It is possible to slow speech and perhaps simplify the task. We know that we should not slow below three movements per second as that will move into closed-loop control (Schmidt & Wrisberg, 2004; Backlin et al., 2008). In addition, numerous researchers have shown that temporal errors (variability) increase with slow movements and that place (spatial target) error increases with faster movements. So whether you slow speech practice depends on the type of error the learner is making. I would use slow speech practice when the child is having trouble hitting targets but not necessarily when the child is having timing or order errors. BUT, I would not slow to fewer than three movements per second because it uses a different control mechanism (closed loop). You can recognize this problem when the normal prosody of the utterance changes.

> ### *Thinking About It*
>
> How do you define the speed movements in speech? Stetson said fundamental unit of speech is the syllable. We know that the temporal relationships between transitions and the vowel, voice onset time, the relative lengths of sounds within syllables, and the relative lengths of syllables are critical components of speech perception and prosody. Therefore, I would not practice at a speech rate that is so low that it changes any of those aspects.

Another area of complexity is the length of the practice stimulus. Thus, perhaps we can break down longer motor tasks into shorter ones. Research has consistently shown that the more loosely coupled movements are the easier it is to break them apart and practice them in isolation. For example, in tennis the serving ball toss is coupled to the actual serving motion but not so tightly that it is unreasonable to practice tossing. On the other hand, the hip rotation and arm swing of the serve are closely coupled during serving and not easily practiced separately. In speech, we have sentences, phrases, words, syllables, and phonemes. Starting with Stetson (1951) many researchers have proposed that the syllable is the fundamental unit of speech. In fact, it is clearly observable that stop consonants do not exist outside the transitions within the preceding or following vowel. In my opinion, speech sounds (phonemes) are so tightly coupled within syllables that they do really exist outside of a syllable. The coupling becomes less across syllables and even less across words and phrases. Consequently, all MLG speech practice takes place at least at the syllable level.

> ### *Thinking About It*
>
> The notion of coupling has clear implications for clinicians trying to figure out the length of a motor program. For speech I would say minimum a syllable. However, there is considerable evidence that speech motor programming can be in elements considerably longer than a syllable. For example, two investigations of the effect on phrase length of inhibition of short and longer phrases clearly demonstrated that speakers, including young children, program across several syllables (Anderson, Meuting, Woolston, & Hageman, 2011; Backlin et al., 2008). Carr (2004) also demonstrated open- and closed-loop control differences across syllables in speech rate tasks.

Although not necessarily directly related to simplification, during prepractice, imagining the movement is useful. Experts in golf and many other sports have reported that visualization of the motor act promotes better performance. Schmidt and Wrisberg (2004) reported research, which suggests that the act of calling up the program is beneficial to learning even when the act is not completed. When the child is old enough, we have begun using "imagination" or auditorization of a successful production of the target before random practice trials. We have not explored this technique systematically, but we assume that speech motor control is similar enough to nonspeech motor control to have positive consequences. Clearly there is more work to do.

Summary

Several variables have been described that are known to affect motor learning for nonspeech activities and some speech activities. We have also proposed certain other aspects of motor practice that improve nonspeech motor control and extrapolated them to speech motor practice. What follows are several examples of utilizing this information to create practice guidelines and hierarchies.

References

Anderson, K., Mueting, E., Woolston, L., & Hageman, C. (2011). *Reliability, accuracy and refractoriness of a transit reaction reaction: Replication with speech in children.* Presentation at the Annual Meeting of the American Speech-Language-Hearing Association, San Diego, CA.

Backlin, J., Corbett, A., Halbur, T., Gaughan, L., Howard, L., Williamson, C., & Hageman, C. F. (2008). *Reliability, accuracy and refractoriness of a transit reaction: Replication with speech.* Presentation at the Annual Meeting of the American Speech-Language-Hearing Association, Chicago, IL.

Carr, L. (2004). *Temporal stability of speech motor programs in young children.* Unpublished Master's research, University of Northern Iowa.

Gaughan, L., Howard, L., & Hageman, C. F. (2009). *Speech inhibition in aphasia: A measure of motor speech programs.* Presentation at the Annual Meeting of the American Speech-Language-Hearing Association, New Orleans, LA.

Guadagnoli, M. A., & Lee, T. D. (2004). Challenge point: A framework for conceptualizing the effects of various practice conditions in motor learning. *Journal of Motor Behavior, 36*(2), 212–224.

Hageman, C. F., Meuller, M., Burda, A., & Bleile, K. (2004). *A motor learning guided approach to the treatment of developmental apraxia of speech.* The 10th Symposium of the International Clinical Phonetics and Linguistics Association, Lafayette, LA.

Hall, P. K., Jordan, L. S., & Robin, D. A. (1993). *Developmental apraxia of speech: Theory and clinical practice.* Austin, TX: Pro-Ed.

Kahneman, D. (1973). *Attention and effort.* Englewood Cliffs, NJ: Prentice-Hall.

Kim, I., LaPointe, L. L., & Stierwalt, J. A. (2012). The effect of feedback and practice on the acquisition of novel speech behaviors. *American Journal of Speech-Language Pathology, 21*, 89–100.

Maas, E., Robin, D. A., Austermann Hula, S. N., Freedman, S. E., Wulf, G., Ballard, K. J., & Schmidt, R. A. (2008). Principles of motor learning in treatment of motor speech disorders. *American Journal of Speech-Language Pathology, 17*, 277–298.

Netsell, R. (1991). *A neurobiologic view of speech production and the dysarthrias.* San Diego, CA: Singular.

Robin, D. A., Jacks, A., Hageman, C., Clark, H. M., & Woodworth, G. (2008). Visuomotor tracking abilities of speakers with apraxia of speech or conduction aphasia. *Brain and Language, 106*(2), 98–106

Schmidt, R. A. (1988). *Motor control and learning: A behavioral emphasis.* Champaign, IL: Human Kinetics.

Schmidt, R. A., & Wrisberg, C. A. (2004). *Motor learning and performance: A problem-based learning approach* (3rd ed.). Champaign, IL: Human Kinetics.

Stetson, R. H. (1951). *Motor phonetics: A study of speech movements in action* (2nd ed.). Amsterdam, Netherlands: North-Holland.

Steinhauer, K., & Preston Grayhack, J. (2000). The role of knowledge of results in performance and learning of a voice motor task. *Journal of Voice, 14*(2), 137–145.

Wambaugh, J. L., Kalinyak-Flizzar, M. M., West, J. E., & Doyle, P. J. (1998). Effects of treatment for sound errors in apraxia of speech and aphasia. *Journal of Speech, Language, and Hearing Research, 41*, 725–743.

Wulf, G., Shea, C. H., & McNevin, N. H. (2003). Increasing the distance of an external focus of attention enhances learning. *Psychological Research, 67*, 22–29. doi:10/1007/s00426-002-0093-6

Appendix A

Language Activities

Therapy seeks to make a treatment sound into a student's regular way of talking. Language and school-based activities help ensure that what is learned in therapy is used in the "real world." This appendix lists 35 language activities. Language activity forms are contained in the accompanying DVD.

Language activities are divided according to whether their primary focus is to facilitate awareness or to practice speech production. The list of activities is illustrative and should be modified, added to, and deleted based on a clinician's interests and philosophy. Most language activities can be carried out either by clinicians, aides, or families.

The following speech activity illustrates some possible ways an activity might be varied. The activity is:

Have the student make a book of words or pictures, each containing the treatment sound, and then say each word to you.

A few of many possible variations include:

1. Make it an awareness activity by removing the speech component and having the student make a book of words or pictures containing the treatment sound.
2. Make it a group activity in which the student shows the book to other students, or make a home activity in which the student and a family member make the book and practice the words.
3. For a younger student, instead of a book of words or pictures find objects whose names contain the treatment sound, and then hide them around a room for the student to find and name. For an older student, replace the book with stories, homework assignments, magazine articles, or newspaper articles.

Language activities for speech may be easily modified by changing the instructions in the following ways:

1. **Imitation:** To create an imitation exercise, have the student repeat the word after you.
2. **Minimal Pairs:** To create a minimal pairs exercise, have the student first say the word with the treatment sound, then say the rhyming word, and then say the word with the treatment sound.
3. **Deletion:** To create a deletion exercise, have the student first say the word with the treatment sound, then without the treatment sound, and then with the treatment sound.
4. **Self-Correction:** To create a self-correction exercise, have the student say the word three times, self-correcting if errors in the treatment sound occur.
5. **Old Way/New Way:** To create an old way/new way exercise, have the student say the word the new way, the old way, and then the new way again.
6. **Similar Sound:** To create a similar sound exercise, have the student first say the word with the treatment sound, then with the most similar sound the student can make, and then with the treatment sound again.

Awareness Activities

1. Read aloud from a book, having the student listen and raise a hand, clap, or ring a bell, whenever a word containing the treatment sound is heard. An easy variation is to tell a story aloud rather than read aloud from a book.
2. Ask a student to silently read a newspaper or story and then circle or write down words that contain the treatment sound.
3. Read a story to a therapy group, having the students compete to be the first to raise their hand when they hear the treatment sound.
4. Read a story to the student and a stuffed animal, having the two "compete" for who raises a hand first when a treatment sound is heard. Let the stuffed animal often give the wrong answer and have the student correct it.
5. Create minimal pairs using household objects or school materials (e.g., wing/ring, light/write). Then say a minimal pair, and ask the student which word (first or second) contains the treatment sound.
6. Tape-record several word lists and ask the student to rate them as being either the new way or the old way of producing the treatment sound.
7. Read paragraphs from stories to the student and occasionally mispronounce the treatment sound (e.g., "Once upon a time there was a printheth who lived in a cathle.") Have the student raise a hand whenever the treatment sound is mispronounced.
8. Make up and read silly stories/sentences that contain the treatment sound produced the "old" way (e.g., "He gave her a diamond wing."). Draw silly pictures to match the silly sentences.

9. In therapy group have a student who can pronounce the treatment sound read sentences aloud, sometimes saying the treatment sound correctly and other times incorrectly. The student with difficulty on the treatment sound does a thumb up/thumb down, depending on whether the treatment sound is correct or not.

10. Work with the student to make a book of words, each containing the treatment sound. An easy variation is to have the student find pictures depicting objects that contain the treatment sound and then have the student paste the pictures into the book.

Speech Activities

1. Ask the student to read a story or article and to say each word that contains the treatment sound.

2. Create a therapy group containing some students who can pronounce a treatment sound and others who cannot. Either read aloud or tell a story to the group, asking the students to listen for the treatment sound and having a student who can pronounce it do so every time it occurs. Ask the student who cannot pronounce it say it after the student who can.

3. Give the student a printed story that has a sticker over words that contain the treatment sound. Ask the student to read the story aloud and "to guess" at the words under the stickers.

4. Read the student a story, stopping at words that contain the treatment sound. The student then says the word. For younger students, have a puppet or stuffed animal tell the story.

5. For a younger student find cards or objects that contain the treatment sound. Place them around a room, turn off the lights, and give the student a flashlight. The student then finds the cards or objects, and says them as they are found.

6. Have the student make a book of words or pictures, each containing the treatment sound, and then say each word to you.

7. Play a board game and adapt the rules to make it a therapy tool (e.g., Move ahead two spaces with an accurate production, Go back one space with an "old way" production.)

8. Use checkers with words containing the treatment sound attached to the back. Have the student say the word taped on the back before moving a piece.

9. Adapt familiar song tunes to include treatment sounds and words (e.g., Larry had a little lamb.)

10. Have the student make a collage with pictures containing the treatment sound, and then name the pictures.

11. Have the student collect and name pictures of friends/teachers who have treatment sound in their names.

12. Have the student write a letter to someone (family/friends) using words with the treatment sounds as many times as possible.
13. Ask the student to list all the toys, animals, foods, and so forth that contain the treatment sound.
14. Have the student look through spelling words, classroom vocabulary words, and reading group books, to find as many words as possible that contain the treatment sound.
15. Have the student substitute the treatment sound for another sound in words in stories or books (e.g., pronounce *polled* as *rolled*).
16. Ask the student to fill in the correct treatment word in sentences either from a bank of words or have the student choose his or her own words.
17. Make up sentences for the student containing words with the treatment sounds for the student to say. Alternatively, ask the student to make up the sentences.
18. Place a word or picture containing the treatment sound on a card, make two copies of each card, and play "Go Fish."
19. Tell the student a story containing words with the treatment sound, and then have the student retell the story to you.
20. For a student who likes jokes, you and the student develop tongue twisters containing the treatment sound.
21. Create a scavenger hunt using words containing the treatment sound.
22. Have the student say a word in a book with the treatment sound, then say it without it, then with it again (e.g., rain, -ain, rain).
23. For a younger student, set toys containing the treatment sound around the room. Blindfold a stuffed animal and have the student tell it the name of the toys.
24. Lay out picture sequence cards that contain the treatment sound and ask the student to tell you the story.
25. Adapt a song to make a silly version containing the treatment sound (e.g., "Christmas is coming, a rooster ate a rat.")

Acknowledgment: The following clinicians and students kindly contributed ideas to this Appendix: Diane Highnam, Lindsay Deitloff, Jill Jensen, Kayla Jiskoot, and Abby Sievers.

Appendix B

Tips for Students

Many students have used this book's resources, often teaching the author as much or more than they were taught. The following ideas are based on helping students learn to work on late-acquired sounds. They are offered as suggestions to beginning students, and are organized into three topics:

1. Resources: A quick guide to how the resources typically are used in treatment
2. Human variables: Nonlinguistic factors that influence treatment
3. Speech practice: Suggestions for practicing speech during therapy

Guide to Resources

Evaluation

An initial screening helps indicate if a student has a speech difficulty affecting a late-acquired sound.

Screening for stimulability helps determine if a student has the capacity to pronounce a sound.

The definition helps decide how a sound should be produced.

Age of acquisition helps in making a decision regarding which sound to teach.

Relative frequency helps in making a decision regarding which sound to teach.

Errors help in making a decision regarding which sound to teach.

Treatment

Metaphors help label a treatment sound.

Touch cues help label a treatment sound through modalities of touch and sight.

Demonstrations show a student how a treatment sound is produced.

Phonetic placement and shaping techniques help establish a sound in a student's speech repertoire.

Key environments suggest which phonetic positions may facilitate pronunciation of a treatment sound.

Word lists are a basis for activities involving words, minimal pairs, deletions, and themes.

Speech exercises help a student to gain experience pronouncing a treatment sound.

Language activities help a student practice a treatment sound using real-world activities and resources.

Human Variables

Recipes: No single therapy technique is right for everyone. Instead of having "one recipe for all occasions," think of therapy techniques as an index box filled with ideas that you select from, add to, and modify to fit the needs of an individual student.

Functional activities: One functional activity is worth a hundred games. Books, class assignments, and newspapers are just a few materials that facilitate learning while facilitating speech.

Let a student know why he or she is there: Talk openly and respectfully to a student about his or her speech. A student needs to understand why he or she is in therapy in order to improve. Don't let a student's speech difficulty become "the elephant in the room" that no one mentions.

Success: A student needs to feel success. In general, if a student is not successful from 50% to 70% on a particular activity, consider changing the activity.

Keep it fun: Be interesting and energetic in therapy. If you have fun, a student is more apt to have fun, too. But while having fun, remember games and entertaining activities are tools, and that the purpose of therapy is to improve a student's speech.

Practicing Speech

Speed: Avoid having a student practice speech by saying sounds and words very slowly. Extremely slow speech employs feedback mechanisms not typically used in speech.

Vowels: Whenever possible, practice consonants in the context of vowels. In everyday conversations consonants are seldom spoken in isolation.

From Words to Conversation: When possible, work on a treatment sound from the level of words to conversation. Those levels have functional value to a student, their use promotes generalization because they are spoken both in and outside therapy, and they appear to be units of motor planning.

Self-monitoring: Promote self-monitoring by not providing constant feedback. Rather than being the monitoring system, encourage a student to monitor his or her own speech.

Self-correction: Provide opportunities for self-correction. Help a student become aware of and correct their own speech.

Communicative value: Help a student learn about the communicative value of a treatment sound through frequent use of minimal pairs, deletions, self corrections, old way/new, and similar sounds.

Functional activities: Base treatment activities on a student's interests, including when appropriate books, magazines, hobbies, and school or work assignments.

People of importance: Keep people of importance in a student's life informed about therapy and, if appropriate, provide them simple therapy activities in which they can participate.

When to dismiss: Typically, a student should pronounce a treatment sound 90% correctly in short phrases and in conversation before dismissal.

Follow-up: Whenever possible follow up after dismissal to make sure a student has not regressed in his or her speech.

Index

Note: Page numbers in **bold** reference non-text material.